ANXIETY
THE
JOULE THIEF

HOW TO TAKE BACK
CONTROL OF YOUR LIFE

DR. CHERYL MEOLA

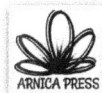

ARNICA PRESS

The material contained in this book has been written for
informational purposes and is not intended as a substitute
for medical advice, nor is it intended to diagnose, treat, cure,
or prevent disease. If you have a medical issue or illness,
consult a qualified physician.

Published by ARNICA PRESS
www.ArnicaPress.com

Cover photo Patricia Kuhn

ISBN: 978-1-7352446-0-0

ANXIETY
THE
JOULE THIEF

HOW TO TAKE BACK
CONTROL OF YOUR LIFE

DR. CHERYL MEOLA

To Christopher and Austin,
who keep me out of my Mind
and living my Life

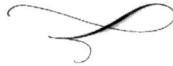

TABLE OF CONTENTS

FOREWORD

IN PURSUIT OF THE WHOLE SAND DOLLAR

The sand dollar story is the heart of my book.
Those broken pieces of sand dollar are coming together in a way
that is helping me help others become whole from their broken pieces.
I see the story like the waves spreading out and the tides rolling in.

Girls' weekend 2016: As a single mom, I didn't get out much without my kids. But I had planned this girls' weekend at the beach for months and was really looking forward to time for *me*. Just me and two of my North Carolina Mom friends, staying at one of their beach homes in Emerald Isle. The beaches down here are warmer and less rocky than where I grew up in New England, and a beach comber's dream. My goal for the weekend was to find a sand dollar for my son. This doesn't seem like the most selfish getaway-goal I could have had. But I am partial to sand dollars–I believe they are my 'spirit animal' or a totem for me to remember the delicateness that survives the ocean's unforgiving currents. So the first night, while my friend chatted away next to me, I walked the beach, searching for that perfect sand dollar to bring home for my little guy.

I didn't find a single sand dollar that evening. Though I searched the beach for almost two miles not one revealed itself in the endless sea of shells. I have no idea what my friend chattered to me about, I was intent in my quest. I didn't notice the beautiful early sunset hues brought out by a stormy beach night floating in, the smells of cresting salt waves around my ankles, or even notice the sharp shells I was walking across in bare feet. Not one sand dollar. Disappointed, I vowed to go out again looking the following day.

The next morning dawned, gorgeous and clear after a night of thunderstorms. The waves had crashed against the beach and created a new seascape. I am not exaggerating when I say there were 10,000 shells and miscellaneous pieces of sea debris washed ashore from the thunderstorm the previous night. I laced up for an early morning run on the beach, expecting to save my sand dollar expedition for after breakfast. Despite expecting the exhilaration of my feet pounding the sand as I ran the beach, I couldn't help but stop every hundred feet or so and pick up a piece of broken sand dollar that jumped out at me while I ran. In all the pieces of sea life washed ashore, they stood out like a neon beacon in the sand.

I frantically picked up the sand dollar fragments and continued to run. I realized I had no pockets or any way to store them, and so I awkwardly thrust my hands out to the sides with the pieces sticking out between my carefully closed fingers. After about a mile, I finally realized how silly I felt running like this, with my hands out and full of broken pieces of shells and sand dollars, running through the uneven sand. I stopped and placed all the pieces of carelessly broken but beautifully worn sand dollars on the shore.

I realized there was so much beauty in these shards, and you could see directly into their broken bodies, the souls of their lives, the weathering of experience on their outer layer mixed with the intricacies and delicateness of their inner matrix. Why can't we see ourselves this way, I thought? Our broken elements are actually windows into our soul showing what we cared about, what we allowed close enough to hurt us, while the rest of our systems continue to hold us up and provide the bones, the structure, that keeps us going. I posted a picture of them, captioning it:

> *Find beauty in broken things*
> *When you love them, they become whole.*

I am the task-oriented overachiever, anxious to control and conquer whatever she set her mind to, who laced up her sneakers that day to run. However, I came back with light pockets and a lighter heart.

I earned this lighter heart by seeing these broken pieces through the eyes of my then six-year-old son. That whole sand dollar that was to be the precious jewel that would make or break my weekend wasn't necessary. It was another goal set upon by worry of not being enough and not achieving enough. I knew he would love these broken pieces exactly the same as if I brought him home a whole sand dollar. That quest for the whole sand dollar, had I not abandoned it for what I had in front of me, would have left me unfulfilled and worried at disappointing my son.

When I got back to the cottage, I kept picking up the broken pieces I had kept, and marveling at their beauty. That morning, I realized, we waste too much of our life looking for the whole and untouched. Meanwhile those beautiful broken pieces are fulfilling all our needs. We just need to realize that they are beautiful without all their pieces. That no amount of worry, or energy, will put them back the way they were, and that the way they are now is whole—just different, and with a bigger story to tell. Now, when I look at a piece of sand dollar, I can close my eyes and visualize its story, and how it came to that way, and how beautiful the story of that piece can be. I do not suffer or waste energy on visualizing finding a whole one anymore.

INTRODUCTION

HOW TO USE THIS BOOK

If you have picked up this book, you are probably stressed in some way. Chances are you have spent an excessive amount of time worrying about something as small as the way a person looked at you at the grocery store to something big like your family's health or financial stability. And chances are you've caught yourself worrying about worrying too much. Have you ever asked yourself "Why do I feel this way?" or "Why I am so stressed? What's the matter with me?"

Stress is a part of everyone's life. We all experience stressors, just in different ways. Stressors can steal away our time and energy from what we really care about—if we let them. And in this overstimulating era that we live in, it is easy to get swept away in worries: *Am I doing enough? Successful enough? Independent enough? Am I too fat? Broke? Not successful enough? Not eating clean enough? Not faithful to my religion?* We can spiral down into this place of reaching for things to worry about without even knowing how we got there. This is when stress becomes anxiety- the constant worrying about an overwhelming amount of things at once.

Anxiety is not our enemy.

Anxiety is what happens when we put too much energy into stressors that are out of our control. What was meant to be a temporary response to an external stressor becomes our "normal" way of reacting to things. We immediately read too much into what is going on around us. What people say to us and about us is a common place we get stuck. Often the worry comes full circle and we start worrying about why we worry too much.

If you have tried therapy for anxiety, you are often told anxiety can be eliminated through cognitive behavioral therapy, mindfulness, or other common practices. What happens though, is at some point, you will have stressors pile on and anxiety will raise its head again. Here we will work on how to move from a fear-based state of worry fear-based to an empowered state of action and strength.

> ANXIETY *is an emotion characterized by feelings of tension, worried thoughts and physical changes like increased blood pressure.*
>
> *People with anxiety disorders usually have recurring intrusive thoughts or concerns.*
>
> *They may avoid certain situations out of worry. They may also have physical symptoms such as sweating, trembling, dizziness or a rapid heartbeat.*
> *(APA, 2020)[1]*

Anxiety is not our enemy.

Anxiety is our body's stress response on never-ending replay. It steals our Energy Joules (a unit of energy in the International System of Units) away from things we care about. This makes anxiety our biggest Joule Thief. It does not think those things should be important when we are "not safe." Learning to work through this fear-based response, rather than avoid it, and replace it with a strength-based response will help us take back our energy joules and spend them where we deem important.

We do not need to "rid ourselves" of anxiety in order to "get better." We need to learn to control our anxiety so it functions as a mechanism of what it really is—an alert system. Not a control system.

This book will help you stop fighting your own survival mechanisms and start actively diminishing the power these mechanisms have over your life. We need to steal back our energy joules from the one thief that matters most: anxiety.

How Did We All Get So Anxious, Anyway?

Anxiety is your body's response to any perceived threat. The result can look like cold sweats; fast, shallow breathing; fatigue or restlessness; or even symptoms resembling a heart attack. Anxiety can cause a hypervigilance with allowing people to connect with you or with trying new things. Anxiety can also cause unexplained irritability and even anger, feelings of impending doom, or intrusive thoughts. If anxiety is present long term, you may start to make different choices in your life. For example, you may decide to take fewer risks, cut out certain parts of your life that make you feel vulnerable, or stay in a job or relationship that is not fulfilling.

Anxiety has become a disorder known to many. It can rear up in many forms- in social situations, as irrational thoughts, in the form of over-compensation, indecision, an inability to leave the house, leave a job, sleep and eating issues. The list goes on.

But anxiety is not the enemy. Going back thousands of years ago, stress was an indicator of a threat to our survival. Humans reacted and then moved on with their life. People were deeply connected to those around them for survival, those who fended for themselves died at the hands of the predator. Humans were not the top of the food chain. Now, we still have those same instincts: to survive and to connect.

Well, look at our world today. "Survival" has been determined as so much more than if you're simply alive. We shouldn't ask ourselves, "Does that trail ahead look like it might lead to a food source, or does it look like a trap with predators?" Simple question, two options. Our choices and expectations have become vast and unattainable. We are more prone to ask ourselves questions about reaching societal goals and being successful than actual survival. Our new go to questions should be:

Are you wealthy?

What do you look like?

Do you fit the profile for success?

What is your title?

What have you accomplished?

How many activities are your kids involved in?

Did you eat "clean" for dinner yesterday?

Do you drive the right car?

. . . the madness goes on.

The second instinct is connection. How do we stay connected? In very disconnecting ways. Through being on our phones in the same room as our loved ones who are also on their phone. Working out in gyms with our headphones on, walking down the street with our eyes on our phone. It feels harder to find places to connect. It's almost a chore. But connection is an instinct in the very essence of our body and soul- it is a survival instinct just like anxiety is a warning of a threat to our survival. Yet we may be afraid to go to a gathering of new people because they will judge us on all those above factors and more:

Do I measure up?

This one question can form all sorts of specific thoughts for us:

What if my mom finds out what I did?

This hurricane sounds really bad. I better go buy forty-seven loaves of bread and every water bottle in the store or else someone will be more prepared than me.

What if someone can tell I haven't showered yet today?

Did my boyfriend just check out that younger girl over there?

I better stop and see my mom. I've only gone to see her once today and she's going to be lonely and wondering where I am.

You get the picture. These, my friends, are Joule Thieves. These little thoughts that cause us to change our expectations of the day's events from exciting and new to safe and stressful. We will talk more about the origins of my affectionate term for these soul suckers in Chapter Two.

TOO MANY CHOICES

One reason so many people struggle with anxiety in our modern society is choice. We have so MANY choices. More often than not, those who qualify as "anxious" are not confronted with a scarcity of resources. They are confronted with an inordinate amount of choices. On top of choice, there is constant stimulation, causing us trouble with focus and decision making. Imagine the quiet, relaxing feeling of sitting on a balcony, overlooking nature–no phone buzzing, no tv talk in the background, just quiet relaxation and, if desired, companionship.

Now think of the scenery we spend most of our lives in–we are inundated with ideas of how to spend our time better, how to look better, eat better. We can stream any movie, television show, or song we want to when we want to, or head out to a store for whatever type of food we're in the mood for. The more decisions we have, and the more information we're exposed to telling us what we need to do better, the more that reptilian part of our brain works. With constant stimulation, we rarely have time to unwind, uncoil that spring inside our brain, and relax. The evolution of our brain has not caught up to our revolution in technology and excess.

Although a large percentage of our population struggles with anxiety, this does not necessarily qualify every one of those people as having an anxiety disorder. A disorder occurs when anxiety is affecting functioning in areas of your life where you functioned healthily before. Anxiety can be the result of another disorder (such as depression, bereavement, or post-traumatic stress disorder). It can be situational, depending on stressors in your life right now; or life transitions; or a result of trauma or suffering from PTSD. Social anxiety. Or another phobia. Anxiety can also be situational and crop up in response to new stressors in your life.

There are millions of ways anxiety shows up in this modern, chaotic, busy world, where society doesn't support slowing down and taking the time to do the things you need to do—that anyone, absolutely anyone, can become a victim of their own thoughts. And that's what anxiety is. You basically become a prisoner of your own "what if" and "why can't I" and "what should" and maybe I should just. . . (do you see how this spirals into things like depression, suicide, and mass shootings?)

If the things in this book don't seem to resonate or help you, that does not mean that you have no other course of action. Anxiety can be secondary to other trauma that may need healing first. For those whose anxiety is very thought-based, controlling is easier than if it lives in your body due to trauma. Even obsessive compulsive disorder (OCD), another type of mental health disorder, is not often treated successfully solely with cognitive or experiential therapy. This book may help, but you may need additional support if your anxiety is trauma-based.

So How is This Book Going to Help?

It might feel like if all you could do was decrease your anxiety, or make it go away with one pill or swipe of a wand, you would be happy. You would be in control. But anxiety isn't the problem. The problem is the way we are managing anxiety. So what's the difference?

Let's try to see anxiety as an overcompensating friend. This friend tries to micromanage everything for us. She/he tells us not to take risks: She/he says: *Don't quit your job and follow your dreams. Don't get that new car. Don't think you know more than me.* Have you ever had a friend like that?

Anxiety is like that friend just moved in and became a permanent roommate—one who nags and warns you of the risks of anything worth living for. Good ol' anxiety comes up with every possible scenario it can to help us be ready for the unknown and unmanageable. It's that piece of our brain we share with reptiles and mammals that wants to, above all us, keep us safe.

A client I worked with used to refer to her anxiety as Phil, an overactive hamster without much to do. We discussed how to build Phil a cage, with lots of productive things to amuse him. When she had something she really needed to focus on, she would put Phil up on his exercise wheel, and feel like she was in control. And Phil was a very productive little hamster when he was managed. Phil is an example of managing anxiety and learning to live with that overcompensating part of our brain. Remember, he's just there to keep us safe, from *his* perspective.

Phil is a good example of how we try to treat the disorder in our mind as a friend or as something we need to take care of, and not the enemy. This book will provide a formula for how to do that. You will learn to take control of your anxiety and how to nurture it into something that can become an asset in times of needs.

This book also provides you with a set of tools, referred to as mindset interventions, to help you see anxiety as something that happens within you but does not control you. I want you to understand what you're dealing with and discover what natural abilities you already possess to help you stay in control of your life. Together we will minimize anxiety's impact on your daily life and make sure your energy is spent on things you care about, rather than over-worrying.

So I hope you get your notebook out and take down some ideas, and mold them into something that works for you. I would say that there is no one formula that works for everyone, but if there's something close, then this is it. Feel free to adapt to what works for you. Then send me some emails and let me know what's helpful and what you changed to make it work for you.

The book gives an eight-week approach to begin the process of taking back control of our lives from anxiety and putting our energy to good use. While you don't have to do this whole book in eight weeks, it does help to have a timeline. For each of the eight weeks, there is a theme and three activities to help you restructure your brain and your life to reach your goals.

Now, I know how your anxious brain is working.

This is going to be three activities for each chapter, that's twenty-four activities I have to incorporate into my daily life in order to beat anxiety? I'm already having a panic attack.

I promise, you calm those hyper neurons. Let them know, *it's okay, I would never do that to you.* There are different places where your coping skills are deficient, and other places they're really strong, or you wouldn't be here, competent enough to read this book. This book is to figure out where your strengths are, identify places you would like to grow, and figure out what will work for you in terms of restructuring your daily life. You can skim some chapters or stop and take notes. You can try all three activities in each chapter, or just pick one. Maybe sit down and look through the table of contents and make a plan of attack before jumping in.

REFRAME, RETRAIN, AND RE-ENGAGE:
THE FORMULA FOR GAINING BACK CONTROL

Often in therapy we talk about working from a "top down" approach (think cognitive behavioral therapy) where we restructure our thinking to fix our body's reaction to external events. Then there is the "bottom up" approach. This is about working on controlling our body's reactions to things in order to tame our wild thoughts and worries. The exercises in this book will come from both sides each week. This is partially because different people learn different ways and have different strengths. My philosophy is that if you work a bit on both simultaneously, you will get the best results as your body and mind start working together to create more peace and balance within. The formula I use to organize activities over the eight weeks in a way that touches both of these strategies is this:

REFRAME + RETRAIN + RE-ENGAGE = CHANGE

REFRAME: The reframe starts with recognizing our common thought patterns occurring. Then we decide what we want to keep and what isn't helpful to us anymore. You may have been bullied in high school and learned to be wary of initiating certain behaviors that called attention to you. Now you may be in a safer place, yet your brain constantly tells you not to stand out or speak your mind for fear of being targeted. You may have been in an unhealthy romantic partnership where someone betrayed your trust, and now your brain constantly tells you relationships are unsafe and your body freezes up anytime someone you are interested in engages with you. These are all signs that we have scripts running in our brain that we have yet to discard. That's when it is time to write some new scripts in order to live our lives, experience what we want, and try new things.

RETRAIN: Retrain has to do with mindfulness and body awareness. Many of the activities ask you to slow down and pay attention to how your body feels during different times, and to become more conscious of how much control you have over the changes that occur. By practicing mindful awareness of your body, you can begin to learn how your body relaxes and work toward that feeling during times of stress. This can also help us to get out of our heads and back into the present moment in order to enjoy and engage in our surroundings.

RE-ENGAGE: Re-engaging is the experiential piece of this formula. In therapy sessions I often employ artwork, Post-it therapy (pretty much anything with ideas written on movable Post-it notes), or we go out to the farm and practice with the horses. This is about doing things a new way. It's about trying out your scripts or testing your body awareness through use of therapeutic activities, referred to in this book as mindset interventions, that help you practice a new way of engaging with your environment, your worries, and your body.

Putting these all together is a holistic way to establish a new you and a new control of your life that you may have lost a bit along the way.

Your Faithful Guide

As a therapist, I find that no matter what problem is presented to me, there is a worry associated with it. People don't come to therapy because they are not worried about anything. People worry about depression, about going through life transitions, about their past, about their current situation, about their panic attacks, intrusive thoughts, their kids, their loved ones, their dog—I have yet to find one without a worry of some kind. So between my own battles with anxiety and my family members', and the constant influx of new stories and worries I've witnessed through my clients, I decided to do the only thing any good nerd would do—lots of research.

I'm the kind of therapist who likes to research. I have a PhD sorta kinda just for that reason. I love to learn, to see how things work on all these interlocking levels of existence—spiritually, emotionally, rationally, and neurologically. I spend lots of money every year figuring out how and why the brain works. I am also the kind of therapist who spends days looking for just the right dandelion to make a wish on. So how does that make me the right person to write this book? Well, part of it is the story (stories) of my clients. Almost everyone who walks in my door has some sort of inflated worry about something. While there are a select few who say they don't, many are just more aware than others of what their brain is telling them to worry about. Many come in wanting to know how to get rid of their anxiety, or how to improve their coping skills for it, or how to stop having intrusive thoughts, live in the past, etc. etc.

What they learn through the process of therapy is what is sapping their energy and causing the stress and worry in their life. They reassess their core values and re-engage in activities that help them align their lives with these values. This allows them to control the anxiety symptoms that have been usurping their lives and teaches them how to bring that energy into what they really care about. A life lived according to your values, it turns out, is a life well lived. I felt like I kept coming back to these same activities and themes that are causing so many of my client's grief. So I sat down with my Post-its and colored Sharpies and started piecing together a formula that could serve as a guideline for others struggling to regain control of their joules and live a life according to their core values.

As I mentioned, I have had my own personal journey with learning to take back control of my life from my anxiety. Every day there are reminders, some conscious, some that have slowly become subconscious, reminding me to live in the moment and trust my gut. I plan for tomorrow, but I live for right now. At least better than I ever did before.

From time to time, if I'm not careful during times of high stress or transition, anxiety still rears its head and prepares for its own version of *Game of Thrones*. I have learned how to create a positive ending to my episodes, however, and remind myself that anxiety is just a toxic friend who cares too much about my safety and not enough about me living and enjoying my life. I have to nudge the boundaries of our relationship back in place and calmly reassert my position on my own throne.

Now, Back to This Book. . .

Each chapter has an explanation of why it's important, a story of how it came to be, and three activities: two to do in the quietness of your own time and one in the moment to help in times of anxiousness. Each chapter has a component of cognitive, mindfulness, and experiential

If one specific chapter stands out as an "AHA! That's my problem, by all means start there. However, for many of us, the building of these exercises on each other is the best way to maintain long term results. You may find you have specific strengths in certain areas, such as an awareness of your values, or being in touch with your body, that you don't need to put a lot of focus on those chapters, but the wholeness of this approach is really your "almost" guarantee of success. Try out all eight, try the activities in each, and find which ones help you the most. Maybe just two or three stick and you find success in those on a daily basis.

OUR FIRST ACTIVITY!

You are now faced with two choices…change your expectations or your actions. Okay, there's a third choice. Remain the same. But you wouldn't still be reading if that was an option for you. So let's take out one of those Post-its. No need to write anything on this one.

Find a blank space on a wall, a dry erase board, your floor—wherever. And place that Post-it right in the middle of it.

What does it look like to you? What does that Post-it say to you right now?

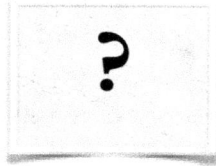

?

That Post-it represents your comfort zone. That's where your anxiety tells you you're ok. All the rest of that blank space? That's life.

That's contentment.

That's happiness.

That's your goals. The rest of your life. Starting now.

The only way to break free of your Post-it Prison is to change your actions or your expectations. If you don't change something about the way you are living your life, then you don't give yourself the opportunity to teach your anxious side that it is okay. That this new thing might be okay. If you are afraid to meet people, to go out and check out a new gym, or bar, or art class, you will NEVER know. Never. You'll only guess. And your anxiety will remain in control.

That's not the kind of uncertainty we want to embrace. The uncertainty we embrace is when we stick our toe through that door to the new experience and know we can't control the outcome. We can only allow ourselves to experience something. You decide if you need to judge it as good or bad. Doing exactly what you are doing now, day in and day out, gives you a 99.9 percent chance of NEVER CHANGING.

Sometimes, action isn't even what we need to change. We may go to work every day, hit up the gym every night, go to art class, meet with your friends, and struggle internally. Every day we put on a face and no one really knows our struggles. They call us stoic, lucky, happy, a role model, but inside we make ourselves sick with worry. Our expectations for ourselves never match up with reality. Our expectations for others are never met. Our expectations for events in our life. So a deeper exploration of our expectations is needed. Where did they start? Who do we know that lives up to them? What is realistic? What would we like to keep as goals that define our core values, and what do we want to discard? We will talk about this in Chapters One and Two.

So. Change your expectations or change your actions. Or remain the same.

At some point, set an alarm on your phone or calendar to go back and track your progress and jot down in the notes section on your progress sheet what surprised you about where you are at now, and how this shifts your goals for the next few days. Also, before this we should write down goals for the next day, week and month. And talk about how it's a process not a flip switch.

CHAPTER ONE

WHAT'S YOUR BEACH MONEY?

My youngest son, Austin, always wakes up as animated as baby lemur at feeding time—man that kid uses his rest well! One morning he was playing around in my bed while I was trying to get a little more shut eye, and he rolls my arm over to look at my forearm tattoo, which is a broken sand dollar.

"Mommy, I just love your beach money picture!" he says to me.

I open one eye and look at him. It's beautiful what kids say, right?

That tattoo has a lot of symbolism for me, and that is why it is on my body in a place I can see regularly. It's a reminder that not all broken sand dollars are mine. Beauty is in the creation of new things from broken ones. Little did Austin know, when he associated "sand dollar" with "beach money," that in some ancient cultures the sand dollar represents mermaid money, or coins from the lost city of Atlantis. To those cultures, the money is something precious and representative of value, much like it has become for me.

When I go through a values exercise, I identify my values as my Beach Money. This is what I hold sacred above all else. Although there has been growth in my choice of words, the core values have basically stayed the same. Instead of family, friends, and pets having separate slots on my values list, they now comprise *Community*. Loyalty and truthfulness have been replaced with *Integrity*. The choice of words matters to me. To me, changing the words represents a transition, or growth. Mindset growth.

WHY ARE CORE VALUES IMPORTANT?

Anxiety comes from living a life that does not match up to a set of expectations. Some of these come from comparing to others, from our loved ones, and from media and society. But the most important expectations we have come from our own core values.

If one of your core values is financial stability, or relationship stability, and you're not experiencing that in your life, then you are going to feel anxious. Or if you think those are the most important things to you and you achieve them and still feel anxious, then a look at what is really important to you may be in order. Perhaps my son wakes up rested every morning because he does not worry about life aligning with his values. Or perhaps when we are young, our values are simple. They are not hidden under layers of confusion.

This chapter has been designed to help you gain a clear understanding of what is most important to you. We will take a look at what takes up your Energy Joules in your life currently. Then we will work toward focusing your energy into manifesting the life you'd like to have according to your core values.

I stumbled across a blog by motivational speaker Scott Mautz that showed a phrase I really love—"Elevate your values to sacred status."[2] The way Mautz talks about values speaks to my heart, and resonates in my work with clients.

"Values are those little things we do each day that exemplify who we are," he writes. "They are the daily little impressions we make that leave a huge permanent impression. You have a choice to live each day in support of your values, or in spite of your values." He points to research that shows most people can rattle off about two values pretty quickly; I've also found this to be true. The issue is that not everyone lets these values guide them. It begs an interesting question:

If you lived your life by your values, without hurting others in the process, would you have regrets?

Values *are* sacred, and hopefully these activities will provoke some deeper soul-searching for what lends meaning to our lives. These values can form a bracket for decision making—do this decision align with what is closest and most precious in my core being? Where would you like to be spending most of your Energy Joules?

At the very least, these exercises will help you identify what your Beach Money looks like, and what other pieces of things that you have been collecting you can safely set down on the beach as you walk home.

ACTIVITY ONE:
WHAT'S YOUR BEACH MONEY?

Materials:

- Several different colored markers

- Several different colored Post-its

- A place to stick them

1. Give yourself at least five quiet minutes to reflect. Focus on the idea of sacred values. Your Beach Money. When you think of a word, image, or phrase that rings true in both your body and mind, write it down on a Post-it. Use a separate Post-It for each one that manifests.

    There's no right answer, or type of answer. There are general values, like integrity, stability, or love, as well as general themes like family, animal rights, or money. You could also do more specific, like my mother, my cat, my bank account. If you get stuck or need inspiration, I've included a list at the back of this book on page 127.

    Play around with words and images as they come, take some notes if you need to, and come up with the word or phrase that best encompasses that value for you. Like I mentioned, *Community* spoke to me more in the later years than *Family* and *Friends*. When you've come up with 3-6 values, put the activity down and take a break. When you come back, see what you want to keep, edit, or delete on your list. I love using Post-its for this reason - they are adaptable and easily replaced or added to at any time.

2. Now, think about where your energy goes on daily basis. Where are some areas you spend energy that are not on your Values Post-its? What stops you from fully participating in your career, your favorite pastimes, being the best p you can be, being the best husband you can be, fighting for animal rights, staying financially stable? From living a life according to your sacred values? Once you figure these out place them on Post-its of a different color. Some examples might be aspects of your job, your family, areas your worry about, physical or emotional pain, fears.

3. Place your values in a designated space. I like to use foam boards, but this could be a piece of paper, a table, poster board, the floor, or some empty space on the wall. The following picture is an example of the space you can use. Place the barriers wherever it makes sense to you on the same board. This will be your Values and Barriers Board. Take some time to look at the results.

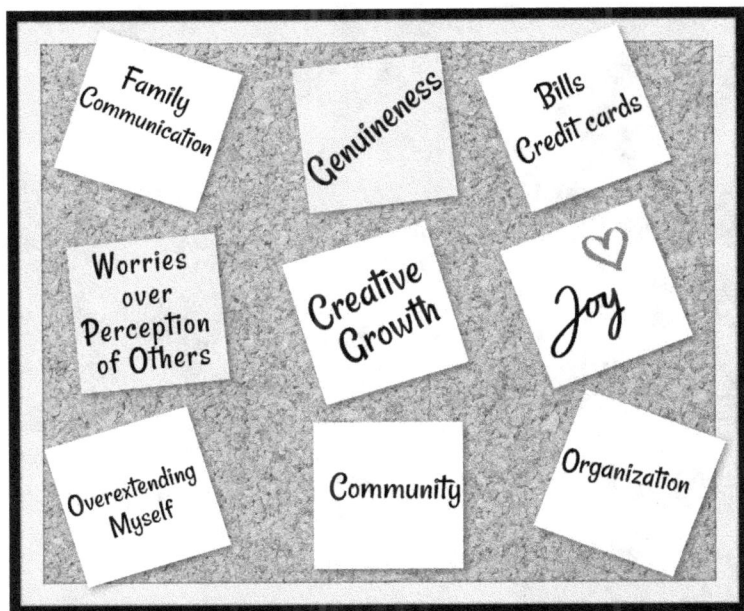

4. REFLECTION

- How are the barriers and values related?

- What stops you from keeping your values sacred?

ACTIVITY TWO:
MONOPOLY STRATEGIES

Materials:

•Whatever you used in the Activity One

1. Give yourself a little break. Maybe twenty minutes, if you're driven and goal oriented. Or give it a few days to sink in. Then go back to the Values and Barriers Board. Spend a few minutes just soaking them in, and then decide if you'd like to move anything around. Okay, you ready? We're going to do a little goal setting next.

2. Have you ever played Monopoly? Some people play solely focused on getting the most expensive properties, Boardwalk and Park Place, and then spending all their money putting hotels there. This strategy leaves them with little left to give when they land on other people's properties. Others buy up as many properties as possible, diversifying gains with hotels, houses, and multiple-colored property monopolies.

Sometimes the purchase of Mediterranean Avenue is the first step in a long line of gains. That's how we're going to set up our goals. If you're a Boardwalk wisher, and that's all you ever want to be, then by all means, set your goal high and reach for it. Most of us will have success by setting up smaller, immediately attainable goals, building upon those goals, and diversifying our energy expenditure.

I've had some success with clients setting up their goals on a foam board in the shape of a Monopoly game like the following picture. They have their values, or ultimate goals for energy expenditure on the Boardwalk and Park Place side of the board. Then they organize the rest of the steps along the way. Some go so far as to use their barriers and create their own chance cards. (Such as: "Mom called—guess I have to go run some errands for her today instead of heading for a walk.")

3. Start with Boardwalk. Where would you like to see yourself in two years? What would a life in which you are holding your core values sacred look like two years from now? Be as specific as possible. If you would like to see yourself with a master's degree in social work, graduating with honors—now there's a start to manifesting your dreams. If your goal is to be back in school, that can be a little harder to break down, but not impossible. Again, try to be as specific as possible! If you send your pal to the grocery store for cheese, who knows what you'll end up with? You send them for the Kerrygold aged gouda, if that's what you want, and you're more likely to receive it! Let's try to approach our life goals the same way! Once you've got the specifics as best you can, make your goals measurable.

    Instead of a goal to be "happy, healthy, and stable," try:

    - "Able to eat what my body tells me to and not binge eat at night."

    - "Able to and actively walk three miles five days a week."

    - "Start dating again, even if it is casually once or twice a month."

    - "Working at the same company in a management position where I make $25K more and can afford to take my dream vacation to Iceland that year."

- "Graduating from a master's program and looking for a job in my field."

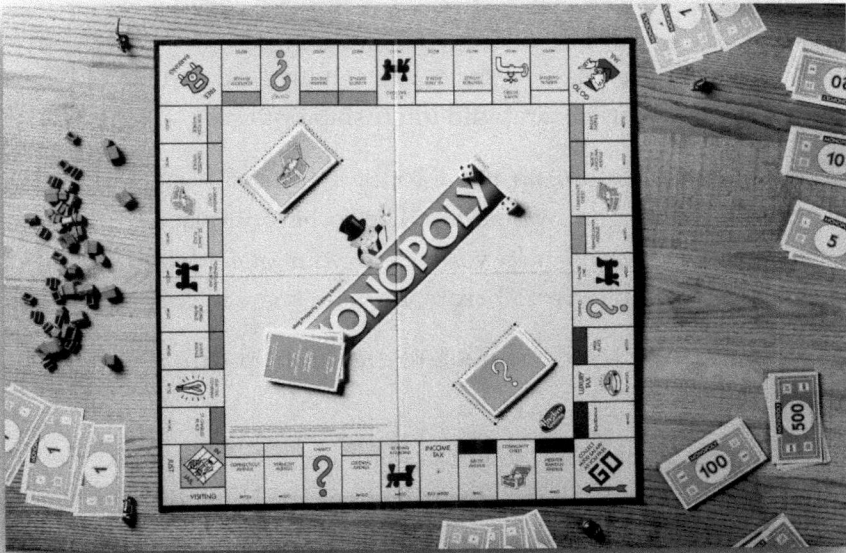

4. Let's head backwards on the Monopoly board a bit from the two years—maybe focus on Atlantic Avenue. What would your life look like one year from now? (Get up and mark that date on a calendar somewhere!) What would you like to have accomplished that will help lead you to your Boardwalk goal? Here are some ideas for one-year goals following the previous examples:

- "Read two books about mindful and intuitive eating and attend yoga and meditation classes twice a week. Have a daily fifteen-minute habit of my own mindful awareness of my body."

- "Walk one mile two days a week, and two miles one day a week, outside of my neighborhood."

- "Start working on myself in therapy before I start dating. Then, begin working on an online profile for a dating site."

- "Take a trip to Iceland."

- "Taken at least half of the courses in my field and be looking at comprehensive exams and internship options."

5. Back up a bit more on that Monopoly Board. Let's hit Virginia Avenue. What goals would you like to have in place two months from now that will help you get to your one-year goal? Staying with our examples from before, here are some ideas:

   - "Purchase at least one book to read to help with my emotional eating."

   - "Attend at least one yoga class and one meditation class locally to try it out. Start a daily five-minute habit of checking in with my body. "

   - "Walk a half-mile to one mile in my neighborhood on one weekend and one weekday per week."

   - "Set up an appointment with a local therapist. Review my goals and see if we will be a good fit."

   - "Write out a plan for trainings I would like to attend in the next year and a cost-versus-gain proposal to my supervisor. Start really focusing on my work with current supervisees to show good management skills."

   - "Come up with realistic budget for saving for Iceland trip."

   - "Started classes at my chosen school."

6. So where does it all begin? What's your Mediterranean Avenue look like? What can you do in the next five days of your life right now to reach that goal?

   - "Track my mood prior to any food I eat and find two new activities for nighttime where I am not binge eating while doing them. Start looking at books online that might help me with my emotional eating"

   - "Write out a schedule for walking this week and enlist my friend to go for a walk this weekend for a half-mile."

   - "Do some research on local therapists. Find one that may specialize in dating or relationship issues. Contact them."

   - "Find twenty minutes to research what I need to do in my career in the next two years to get my promotion. Research trips to Iceland and choose what I'd like to do there."

   - "Contact the school of my choice and schedule a time to talk to an advisor about entrance this fall."

7. You may have no idea where to get started on your board, or how to work your goals backwards in time. Meditate on it. Go for a walk. Bounce ideas off your significant other, a friend, or your pet. Look over past accomplishments that you feel good about. Think about a mentor you've had and aspired to be. Someone who has done what you would like to do or something similar. Contact them and see what it would take for some of their time to work on goal setting or get some ideas. You might be surprised how open some people are about helping you reach similar goals. And if they are not, try someone else—sometimes we meet up with a closed door and give up, when that door was just redirecting us to a better one!

Do whatever will make you feel like you are reaching your goals more fully. You will be on your way to full control of the Monopoly board (aka your life!)

8. REFLECTION: Who do you find most authentic in your life? Go back in time if you have to and think of someone who rang true to your core being - who lived a life according to what they believed in? How do you know they did? What small (or large) change can you make right now in your life to align yourself with your values as they did?

ACTIVITY THREE:
IN THE MOMENT MINDSET SHIFT

Find some time to sit quietly in solitude. Clear your head of the past and current anxieties. Allow them to enter, pass through, and rest. This is their nap time. We are going to spend some time visualizing our future we have laid out for ourselves. Ask yourself these questions as you picture it:

- What do I look like?

- What am I wearing?

- What am I eating/drinking?

- Who am I with?

- What was I thinking about?

- What was I focusing my energy on?

- Wat do my surroundings look like?

- How do they make me feel?

- What do I smell around me?

- What do I hear?

Sit with this and imagine yourself living this life. Breathe deeply into the future you are going to create for yourself.

CHAPTER PROCESSING

Come back to this activity after a break, whether it's an hour, a few days, or whenever works within the week. Look at your board.

Is there anything you'd like to change, add, or subtract? Go for it! This board is yours and we'll use it as a map to guide us in the next chapter. Keep it handy as we talk about our energy spending and our Joule Thieves.

CHAPTER TWO

COUNTING YOUR ENERGY JOULES

Earlier I introduced you to the concept of Energy Joules, the amount of energy you start with each day. In this chapter, we will look at how you spend your Energy Joules. Your Energy Budget, if you will. We will discuss why it's important for us to know where we spend our energy.

Here's the story behind my affectionately named term, Energy Joules.

In my office I keep a partially empty vase. I had the idea of putting fresh flowers in it, but then there's the issue of the maintenance of the flowers and spillage and shedding on the carpet. There are also client allergies to consider. So it's empty except for some tiny round pieces of sea glass that decorate the bottom.

One day, in session with a client, in between sorting out her core values from her current life, I scooped up the sea glass orbs from the bottom of the vase to illustrate where this client was spending her energy in her daily life.

Each little jewel-like orb from the vase represented a unit of energy the client had at the beginning of the day. I was delighted to remember from my high school physics class that a joule was also a unit of energy. So now Energy Joules is how I refer to these orbs.

I explained that energy is a limited resource, just like money. We need to be aware of where we spend our energy just like we need a budget to know where we're allocating our funds. So much of the time, we are spending our energy on things that do not give us anything in return. These energy sucks can be a part of distorted thinking like trying to be a mind reader and figure out what other people are thinking. It can be a toxic relationship (mother, brother, friend, boss, boyfriend, you name it). Or it could be meeting expectations we have set for ourselves that do not align at all with our core values.

ACCESSIBLE ENERGY *is how I refer*
to the energy that can easily be spent.
This can be translated into your level of motivation in the moment.
When I say there are always 100 units tucked away somewhere,
here's how I explain this:
If I was lying on my couch scrolling through social media
and feeling totally demotivated to do anything,
and suddenly I read a status that said
"Heading over to visit my bestie Cheryl M!"
from a friend who I don't see often, I may suddenly spring off the couch,
wash my face and put on a clean shirt and speed clean my entire first
floor (probably pop a breath mint or brush my teeth too!).
That energy was there but a moment ago I couldn't access it.
When properly activated however,
it suddenly becomes usable and accessible in the moment.

While my client was sorting where her energy goes on a daily basis, many of these Energy Joules ended up in the client's barriers column rather than in her values column. When this happens in our lives, we create an energy deficit—just as if we were spending our money on things that offer us nothing long term in return.

I discussed with my client how many energy units she typically starts each day with. We imagined that a typical healthy day starts with 100 units of energy, to make our math easier. We also looked at how some days, if her mental health was dragging her down, she may start your day with sixty units of energy. With depression or dread of an upcoming event, some days she might only start with twenty-five. She may still have her 100 units tucked away somewhere, but on those days, only twenty-five Energy Joules are accessible.

I used to refer to these as our Energy Suckers, until a client coined the term Joule Thieves. I love it. There's nothing I love more than a clever play on words!

We will go through this process shortly ourselves to uncover where our energy may get sucked up on a daily basis. This activity is all about making an investment in yourself. Just like a financial budget, this will really open your eyes to where you are spending all your energy, and what you need to do to re-calibrate your life according to your values.

We've discussed how there are have barriers that stop us from living a values-filled life. Our Joule Thieves—those anxieties that control our decisions (or indecisions) on a daily basis—are often stealing more of our accessible energy than we realize. We have more control over how much these barriers take from us than we realize when we are caught up in our daily thought patterns.

Grab your Values and Barriers Board from Chapter One and let's get budgeting! You, my friend, are about to take back possession of your joules.

ACTIVITY ONE:
YOUR ENERGY INVESTMENT PORTFOLIO

Materials:

- Your Values and Barriers Board

- A writing utensil

1. This activity will focus on how to categorize the barriers you listed into necessary energy suckers and unnecessary joule thieves. Then we will break down how to take back some of our energy and spend it the way we would like, according to our values.

2. Look at your Values and Barriers Board. Organize your Post-its into two categories: *Obligations* and *Optionals*.

    OBLIGATIONS are the unavoidable responsibilities that are physically, mentally, or emotionally draining. Some examples are caring for aging parents, dealing with toxic co-workers, suffering from chronic physical pain, parenting responsibilities, keeping up with housework, and budgeting. These are things that may be draining but are not going away any time soon. Learning to balance the amount of Energy Joules you spend on them becomes a critical life skill for living a values-filled life.

    OPTIONALS are things we put our energy into that we might be able to negotiate in or out of our lives, depending on how much energy we have to spend. Some of these are binge-watching Netflix, oversleeping (or overeating, overmedicating, overindulging), social media, negative thoughts, worrying about

Communication	My Spiritual Growth	Worries about my job	Sleeplessness
Honesty		Money worries	Pressure from other people to do what they think is important
Taking care of my Dog	Being supportive to my Family in all ways	Worries about my Dog's old age and health	Job Review at work next week

Communication	My Spiritual Growth	**OPTIONAL** Worries about my job	**OPTIONAL** Sleeplessness
Honesty		**OPTIONAL** Money worries	**OPTIONAL** Pressure from other people to do what they think is important
Taking care of my Dog	Being supportive to my Family in all ways	**OPTIONAL** Worries about my Dog's old age and health	**OBLIGATION** Job Review at work next week

what others think of you, toxic friendships or relationships, over-extending yourself by volunteering your time for too many things, giving of yourself in too many places, or just spending all your time doing and none of it being. These are general examples and your list may look very different from someone else's. Some things a person lists as *Optionals* may be *Obligations* to you.

> *Every time I find myself putting energy into*
> ### PRESSURE FROM OTHER PEOPLE
> ### TO DO WHAT THEY THINK IS IMPORTANT,
> *I will stop and say out loud:*
> *"You are not getting my energy today.*
> *Instead, I am putting my energy into*
> ### BEING SUPPORTIVE TO MY FAMILY IN ALL WAYS."

Some questions to help yourself organize:

• If you're unsure where an activity, person, or worry belongs, close your eyes and think about how you feel directly after doing this activity or interacting with this person. Do you feel recharged? Do you feel numb? Exhausted? Are you more motivated or less? This can help you categorize into one or the other category.

• What would your life look like without this activity? Close your eyes for a minute and picture yourself, going throughout your day, without this activity or relationship existing.

• What feelings come up for you when you picture this?

ACTIVITY TWO:
LAY OUT YOUR JOULES

Materials:

- Your Values and Barriers Board

- Something to represent your 100 Energy Joules (coins, seashells, M&Ms, rocks, etc.)

1. Take out whatever you chose to represent your Energy Joules you start with each day. Spend them out like you would on a typical day for you. For example, if you start with 100 joules, you may put twenty into your Value of "caring for my pets," and ten into "family" because you call your mom every morning on the way to work, and fifty into work, and five into health because you ate food but you don't know what or whe n you ate, and fifteen into your value of "self-love" because you read a book for fifteen minutes before going to bed. But that leaves nothing for exercise or competition, which are important to some people. Spread them out as you see best.

2. Take a look at your typical day. Write down any observations you might have about where you spend your energy. At the end of the day, do you generally feel wired? Overwhelmed? Exhausted? Content? Numb? Write down a few sentences about how you feel.

3. Use your cellphone to take a picture of where your Energy Joules are laid out. This will help you remember every time you look at your phone, and we will also use that photo for an activity later on in this book.

ACTIVITY THREE:
ONE JOULE AT A TIME

1. Pick one area in your Energy Joules layout that you would like to remove some joules and place them directly on top of where you would like to spend them instead. How hard was that? How do you think you can manifest that energy change in your life, right now?

2. THIS IS YOUR ENERGY GOAL. Write it down. And then again. Repeat it to yourself. Keep track of your progress in the chart at the back of this book. Tell yourself that this is your goal and you are-worth it!

For an added reminder, write this goal down on a Post-it: Every time I find myself putting energy into (Insert Joule Thief identified), I will stop and say out loud "You are not getting my energy today. Instead I am putting my energy into (Insert value chosen)."

The more energy you put into this mindset shift, the better your brain will listen.

CHAPTER THREE

REPLACING FEAR WITH EMPOWERMENT

Anxiety is a response to something that threatens us. This is a fear-based response that comes hard-wired into our body. You do not have to teach yourself to be afraid of things that cause pain. It can steal your Energy Joules faster than you can say "Run!"

Empowerment is something that gives us strength and offers our Energy Joules renewal. This is a strength-based response. You have to re-wire your brain to come from a place of empowerment instead of fear.

Approaching life from an empowered perspective allows us to live a more values-filled life. This approach is necessary to focus our energy on the activities, people, and ideals that give us back as much as we put in. Even the happiest and most content of us have unwanted feelings. These feelings may be rooted in fear and worry or may be described as:

- Feeling down in the dumps

- Feeling triggered by external events or people

- Feeling lonely, overstimulated, overwhelmed, underappreciated, or disconnected

- Feeling bored (plenty of evil can happen from boredom!)

All of these feelings can trigger our fear-based response system. By identifying the primary emotion triggered in each situation and learning what we are trying to avoid by being "fearful", we can start

51

to understand our triggers and underlying motivations to worry and fear.

The activities in this chapter are geared to help you keep your energy invested primarily in your priorities, and not in all your *Obligations* and *Optionals*. First let's look at what choices you make when you experience an emotion, and particularly when your fear-based responses are activated. Then we will start the work of re-programming our brain's response to these triggers. Yes, initially we may have a fear-based instinctual reaction, but we can learn to immediately re-route that into a thoughtful, empowered-response.

Part of this process is identifying your "go-to" coping mechanisms. These are typical responses to our fear system being triggered. We will look these go-to mechanisms and categorize them as numbing or energizing. Then, we will decide which ones we would like to keep and which ones we will replace.

Next, we will find a model to help us create goals for positive, empowering mindset interventions to take the place of the coping. Instead of "coping" we will be activating, growing, and moving.

Often I picture the Sand Dollar, with predators abound,
in the depths of the ocean, waves and sand pounding against it.
I picture its slow progress, tentacle by tentacle,
as it moves forward in its journey.
I think about what my little tentacles are-
what holds me in place as discouragement, shaming,
disconnection, and other fear-based symptoms attack me.
Sometimes I feel attacked by predators,
but sometimes it is an internal battle.
I have to spread my tentacles and hold on to what feeds me,
what grounds me, and what offers me stability
through all the waves and sand pounding against me
along the way.

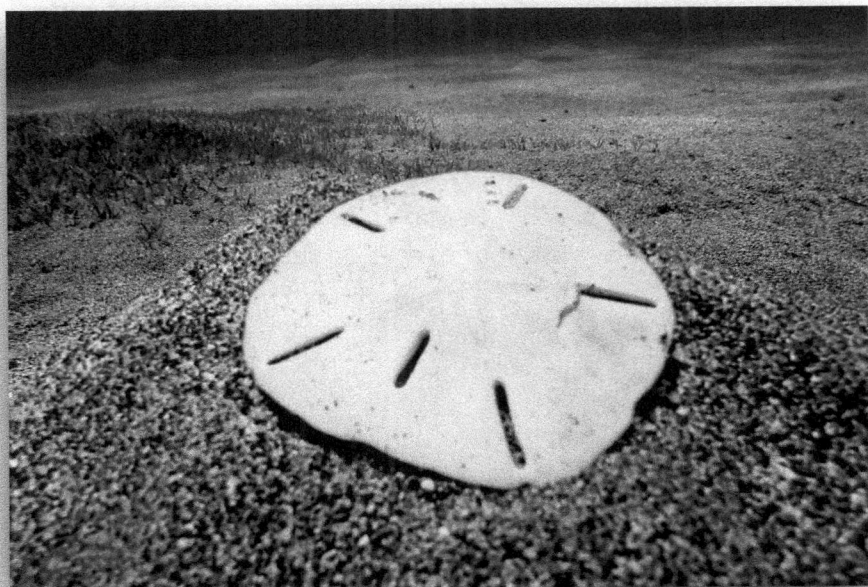

One thing that separates us from those we admire is the "f" word: Fear. Thoughts like:

- *I'm not smart enough* (Or replace smart with any adjective- skinny, pretty, rich, fast, creative, social, etc.)

- *He/She's out of my league*

- *No one will buy into what I say*

- *He/She should be ashamed of him/herself* (Usually has to do with "I" should be ashamed of something)

- *I can't handle this*

These tend to crop up in different ways but have the same underlying message: *I'm not good enough*.

So when we are making life decisions based on a script that says "I'm not good enough," we are only looking at obstacles that make us feel incapable. And scared. The way to start re-writing this script is to start recognizing what we can do. This is empowerment.

Now you've come from a place of fear for a while. It might have been a slow-burn process, growing for years with constant little events piling on the evidence. Perhaps a significant event triggered a faster acceleration of the *I'm not good enough* script. Regardless, it will take a little time to re-write your brain to a default of empowerment instead of fear. This chapter contains some of the first few steps in the re-write process. We'll familiarize ourselves with the steps before we get into the activities.

The first step to empowerment is establishing safety. As many years of horse-handling and training has taught me, if we do not work to establish a safe environment, learning cannot occur. When we feel safe, we can learn, grow, and recognize our strengths, our accomplishments, and our progress. We cannot learn to respond with empowerment when we cannot establish safety. Our fear system will be on standby, waiting for something to trigger it to take over.

In my dissertation research, I looked at whether a one-hour experience with horses could improve the counseling self-efficacy and state anxiety levels in students. Counseling self-efficacy is the positive feelings (or lack there-of) related to competency in starting to see clients that students experience. State anxiety is situational anxiety, not someone's characteristic tendency toward worry. What I had hoped the research would show is that the structured supervision-type experience with the horses would increase the students' counseling self-efficacy and decrease their anxiety about meeting with clients. Most of the counseling students in the study were either in their first semester of meeting clients one-on-one or were starting that process the following semester. What I found out was actually more helpful and revelational than I had hoped. It was an example of replacing fear with empowerment through in-the-moment mindset shifts, much like what we are practicing (without horses!) in the activities here.

The experience did show that the participants' counseling self-efficacy increased significantly higher compared to a control group. However, the state anxiety only showed a slightly smaller decrease than in the control group. There was a qualitative (or written) questionnaire that gave some significance to this finding. Eight of the ten participants in the treatment group discussed how the experience of grooming and then leading the horse was an anxiety provoking situation. They were highly motivated to connect with the horse due to positive feelings toward the animal, but also due to a fear of the animal (either their rejection or a physical fear). For some, having a farm staff member and myself watch the interaction was the anxiety provoking part. Even though what we were asking them was outside of their comfort area, each participant was more motivated to connect with the horse than to quit.

What the participants reported discovering during the leading exercise with the horse was that a fear of losing connection with horse paralleled their worries about beginning work with clients. They were afraid of choosing the wrong signal with the horse, upsetting or misinterpreting the horse. Each participant related these feelings back to their current worries about counseling. What helped their counseling self-efficacy increase, however, was that they had the experience of working through anxiety and still establishing a strong connection with the horse.

Most participants noted that natural coping skills were their "go-to" in these situations. With a counseling client, they may have shut down for fear of judgment or doing something wrong. But with the horse, they felt the need to stay present and connected. Some participants noted that at times they felt they lost the connection with the horse but were able to re-connect by staying present and using some self-identified strength they already possessed. They realized that anxiety in the moment is normal and can happen in session without harm to the therapeutic relationship. Everyone left the sessions feeling they had experienced something positive that would carry over into counseling sessions. Even though they experienced a spike in anxiety during the process, they found a way to approach the challenge from an empowered perspective.

The fears those counseling students faced were transformed from fear-based thoughts to empowered-based thoughts. *I am afraid of this, but I have skills and strengths to overcome that fear, and the outcome will be far better than my worries predicted.*

While I wish I could take you all out to the barn, we are going to do our mindset intervention without horses. We will create an experience that may raise your anxiety while you are in a safe and supportive place. We will recognize what helps you get through that fear and find ways to help you return to that strength-based power when your fear is activated.

ACTIVITY ONE:
CHOOSING EMPOWERMENT OVER FEAR

Materials:

- Writing pad and utensil

1. Start by answering this question: When you would rather not think about your fears, or you are trying to avoid a negative feeling, what do you find yourself doing? Do you find yourself lashing out at others? Binge watching Netflix? Writing a song? Taking a drive in your car? Eating ice cream? Going over lists in your head? Each time you think of a go-to activity for you when you would rather not deal with feelings, write it down.

2. Next, label each activity as *Numbing* or *Energizing*. *Numbing* is a fear-based response to our stressors. Generally, we are numbing to hide from our fears. What do you do when you would rather not deal? Do you carb load? Binge Netflix all night? Sleep? Drink? Facebook? Speed date? Think of the activities you spend time on that makes you feel worse off or less healthy than when you started. These activities waste more Energy Joules without creating any more.

    Energizing activities might distract us from the feelings, but they leave us feeling more motivated and refreshed to tackle our problems. What do you do to escape your feelings that ends up contributing to your well-being? What makes you stop and think after, *wow I'm glad I did that! I feel better!* Is it cooking a healthy dinner? Calling a friend? Reading? Going for a long drive? Exercising? Writing? Think about how you feel afterwards. If in some way you are more able to deal with your stressors, then that activity helped you take back control of some of your Energy Joules.

3.   *Energizing* activities bring us closer to our goals and empower us. Choose something on your energizing list and write it down somewhere you will see it multiple times a day. This might be your planner, the back of your phone case, your dashboard, your mirror, your laptop. Every time you come in contact with the word, give yourself a moment to feel empowered.

4.   Write down something on your *Numbing* list and keep track of how many times you choose this activity for a week. Anytime you feel yourself about to carb-load or mindless scroll your social media, check in with your power word. Say out loud "I have a choice how I spend my energy. Right now, I choose ____."

Anytime you choose your *Energizing* activity over your *Numbing* one, that's a gold star! Check in and write about how you felt before and after your choice. It's okay if you don't always choose empowerment this week. But remember to reward yourself when you do and TRACK YOUR PROGRESS. Use your Values and Barriers Board and literally put a gold star up there for yourself if that is what helps you!

ACTIVITY TWO:
MODELING EMPOWERMENT

WHAT KIND OF LEARNER ARE YOU?

*These mindset interventions work faster when you know
the best way your brain intakes new information.*

*Think back to school or trainings you've attended.
Do you retain the most information from hearing,
seeing, performing, discussing, taking notes?*

*If you're an auditory learner, repeat these empowerment
statements out loud to yourself each day.
Multiple times if needed.*

*Record yourself saying them and listen to them on your way to
work, before picking up your kids from school
or stepping in the door to go home or to an important meeting.*

*Hear yourself believing in yourself.
If it's too hard, ask someone to read them
about you and record that.
Whatever works - again the limit is only your imagination.*

1. Think of someone you admire—someone who lives a life according to their values. This could be your mentor, a person you've seen speak about something important to you, a humanitarian, a leader, a boss, anyone whose qualities you would like to possess. Take some Post-it notes and write down what qualities this person possesses that you would like to have.

2. Now write down at least 10 words to describe yourself. They may be qualities, personal characteristics, (resilient, cautious, nervous) or they may be temporary states (always tired, numb, isolated).

3. Look at the lists. Explore the similarities and differences in your mind. Pick one quality you feel you could actively engage in expanding in yourself. Choose an activity that you can do in the next twenty-four hours that fully incorporates that quality. Now go out and do it!

4. After performing that activity, your anxiety may want to brush aside your success. You may find yourself thinking fear-based statements, like you are a fraud, and one activity does not mean you have obtained the quality you admire. These are all FEAR-based thoughts! Pick one empowered thought and stick with it. Look in the mirror and repeat it to yourself as you smile. Stand in warrior pose if it helps. You OWN this accomplishment.

ACTIVITY THREE:
IN THE MOMENT MINDSET SHIFT:
THE EMBODIMENT OF EMPOWERMENT

Materials:

- Your brain

1. What words or definitions come to mind when you see this word?

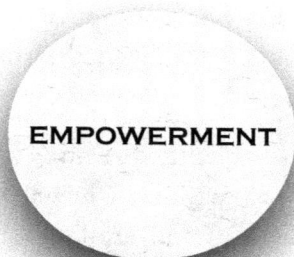

EMPOWERMENT

Take a few moments to picture it. What images come up for you? What does it look it? Where in your body do you feel empowered?

2. What words or definitions come to mind when you see this word?

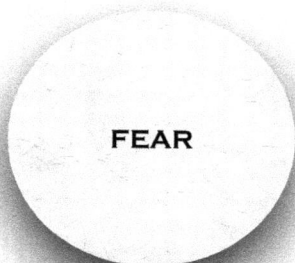

FEAR

Take a few moments to picture it. What images come up for you? What does it look it? Where in your body do you feel fear?

3. Go back to the previous image. Find yourself in that place where your body recognizes and acknowledges fear. Now, slowly, become aware of how different this is than the place of empowerment. Picture yourself facing that fear.

Slowly, change each one of your sensations to reflect that place of empowerment. Focus on each one of your five senses. Go back to what you experienced in empowerment. Change what you are sensing to one of empowerment for you. Do the same for any body part you can sense you are holding fear in. As you start to feel a difference in each body part, in each sensation, focus on it and label the change. Move yourself forward into empowerment as you face that fear.

There. You've done it. You've positioned yourself opposite a fear, and instead of cowering or numbing, you are empowered and doing. You are accepting and moving forward and allowing yourself to be, regardless of the outcome of that once-powerful fear. You are embracing your whole self and unafraid of the judgment, shame, and scrutiny you once placed upon yourself.

Don't worry, I've made you a script.

I have faced my fear of (Fear You Have Faced). I have accepted that this fear is a part of my life story and I choose to create my own story from here on out. I will move and flow with empowerment and grace, regardless of the outcome of this once-powerful Fear. I allow myself to be my whole self and embrace my whole self by being unafraid of judgment, shame and scrutiny of (Fear You Have Faced).

CHAPTER FOUR

DON'T GO WITH THE FLOW, BE THE FLOW

I love this quote by the Chinese philosopher Lao Tzu: "Be like a mountain, but flow like a great river."

How do you create the feeling of being the foundation of your own life while you still allow and even seek things to embrace along the journey?

What does flow look like? Some might call it being "in the zone. [4]" In psychologist Mihaly Csikszentmihalyi's work on happiness and flow, he defines it as "a state in which people are so involved in an activity that nothing else seems to matter; the experience is so enjoyable that people will continue to do it even at great cost, for the sheer sake of doing it." Basically, whatever you choose to do allows you full access to your energy without much effort to do so, you are in a state of flow.

The idea behind this chapter is that we can create a life that is a larger definition of Csikszentmihalyi's flow. We have more control over our lives than we realize. If you stop and categorize every decision you make, you would put them in categories of being intrinsically motivated versus extrinsically motivated. Extrinsically motivated is going with someone else's flow—what makes them feel happy. Intrinsically is making us happy. The more we make intrinsic decisions in our life, the more opportunities we create to experience the definition of flow Csikszentmihalyi described.

The idea is to create your own flow instead of being dragged along by everyone else's.

Before moving completely into my own private practice, I took a chunk of time and money and invested it into a business boot camp for private therapy practices.

One of the first activities we developed was to plan out a perfect day. *What would it look like if we could do whatever we wanted within our job, our life, our existence? How many clients would I see and when? What else would I put energy into?*

At first, I only half-heartedly answered the questions. But after being in practice for a few months, I went back and really invested time in planning out my daily schedule to try and make it as perfect as possible. This was a huge turning point for me. I started to realize that I was living my best life, at that moment, and that any anxiety I was having about work and scheduling was simply my own doing. It was when I stopped going with everyone else's flow and started creating my own flow. If I wanted to be done with work on Thursdays at 1 p.m. to pick up my kids at school dismissal, it would cause me immense stress to have to skip that and see clients until 4 o'clock. I realized that no one was telling me to do this. I was motivated extrinsically, to satisfy their needs while sacrificing my value of being a present mom. I had structured my week to know how many time slots I need filled to pay myself, and I specifically did not make these slots on Thursday afternoons. I was creating my own anxiety trying to accommodate everyone else's happiness. This is what "going with the flow" looks like– going with everyone else's flow.

Are there things that might come along that are worth shifting your flow for? Yes! But this is all about balance and expending energy on things that matter. To you. Every single day.

Well, my friends, here are some activities to do that very thing. I've included a worksheet in the back if you want to use it as a template for Activity One, or you can use your own creativity.

SAND DOLLAR FLOW

The sand dollar has lived its life at sea weathering all sorts of conditions. The ocean throws all sorts of variables at the sand dollar: currents, bottom-feeding predators, sand - so so much sand.
But the sand dollar just tightens up and stands its ground.
And eats up all that sand. Literally. The sand ends up weighing the sand dollar down so they cannot be swayed and moved by the changing currents of the ocean. Pretty cool, huh?
They really known how to create their own flow.

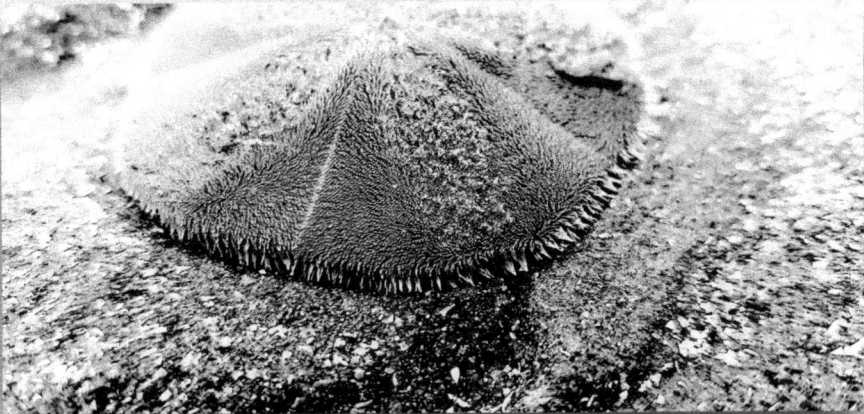

ACTIVITY ONE: CREATE YOUR FLOW:
IMAGINING A VALUES - FILLED DAY

Materials:

- Values and Barriers Board

- Blank paper or worksheet from end of book

- Writing utensil

1. Flip your board over or start with a fresh piece of paper. Make sure to have your Values and Barriers Board handy if you haven't memorized everything on it yet.

We are going to map out the best day you can envision for yourself. The most excellent day you can imagine, without anything crazy or extravagant happening. It's important this vision is just an ordinary day because while winning the lottery or taking an expensive trip would be fabulous, we are working toward you living your best life every single day. This day will show you putting your energy into the things you care about and not letting the energy suckers take anything away from you.

Start with what time you would like to get up in the morning and walk yourself through your whole day until bedtime, either in words or pictures. Be as detailed as you can get. Manifestation is all about the details! Write down what you'd like to have for breakfast, with whom you will eat, what you can wear to work or wherever you are going for that day, through when you settle down for sleep that night.

You can even get into what car you are driving, what the weather is typically like in this perfect place, the scenery, your phone ringtone–take some time and really visualize this Values-Filled Day. Then answer these questions:

A. Where is your energy going on this day? Look at your values again. How much of that day is a life lived according to your values?

B. Look at where you laid out your Energy Joules previously (look at the picture you took). Where do you notice the biggest differences?

C. How do you feel when you think about this being a step on the journey to that Values-Filled Day? Right now, by giving your time to this activity, you are manifesting and creating this Values-Filled Day one Energy Joule at a time!

ACTIVITY TWO:
GET YOUR CREATIVE JUICES FLOWING

Materials:

• Writing utensil and paper or computer

• Your creative juices

1. Sit and think about some of the things we have covered in the past few weeks. Set a timer and prepare to free-write for the next fifteen minutes. During that time, you are allowed to fully process (in full word-vomit style, if necessary) all the learning you have done about yourself and your progress so far. We've learned about what you care about, the ways you spend your energy, and where you desire your energy to go.

    Some things to consider are:

    A. What has helped you the most so far in this process?

    B. What feels like the biggest barrier for you?

    C. If you were to ask the person who you chose in the last chapter as your model, what kind of advice do you think they would give you right now?

These are just prompts if you need somewhere to go, but the point of the exercise is to not stop writing/typing for the full fifteen minutes until the timer goes off, not even for a few seconds. This will allow you to clear through the debris to see what is really lurking underneath.

If you feel up to the challenge, try twenty minutes!

Repeat this activity three times this week.

We are standing up and taking back control of what we put our energy into.

You have it within your grasp!

Don't give up!

ACTIVITY THREE:
MINDSET SHIFT: DETOX TIME

Materials:

- Your lists of *Obligations* and *Optionals*

- A writing utensil

1. Mindset Shift/Re-engage: Take a look at your *Optionals* list from Chapter Two. Choose one item listed that you would like to eventually eliminate or significantly reduce from your energy spending.

   We are going to plan a thirty-day detox from this one thing. Is it Candy Crush? Drinking? Social media? A toxic friend? Dating? Oversleeping? Sugar-loading? Choose whatever applies best for you.

2. Pick a replacement or mindset intervention—a daily habit that can be your go-to whenever you crave this former Joule Thief. Some examples are journaling and tidying up or see the sidebar for more.

3. Write this down for yourself: "Today is (insert date). I am starting my thirty-day detox from (insert choice of energy-sucking Joule Thief). This is a barrier to living my Values-Filled Day and I am committed to working on this day for thirty days. Whenever I feel like adding this Joule Thief back into my life, I will (insert new mindset intervention) instead. I am grateful to have (new mindset intervention) in my life."

FIVE SENSES ACTIVITY

Develop a sense of being present
as your replacement mindset activity.

Take a deep breath and look around you.
Notice FIVE elements in your environment
you have not noticed before.
Be as detailed as you like.

Maybe the patterns of your clothing's fabric, or the way
the color of something changes as the texture changes.

Next, listen for sounds you have not noticed before.
See if you can find at least FOUR.

Take a deep breath and feel the air around you -
what does it feel like?

Think of other things you can feel as you pay attention -
your clothes, the ground beneath you....

Breathe in and become aware of any smells around you.
Any taste.

Take one more deep breath
and enjoy being fully present in your environment.

Anxiety: The Joule Thief by Dr. Cheryl Meola

CHAPTER FIVE

COMPARTMENTALIZING AND PRIORITIZING

Starting to separate who we are from what we worry about is the hardest part of this entire process. For many people with anxiety, compartmentalizing is a difficult concept. Thoughts and worries have become so tangled up in the concept of self that they almost define themselves by what they are afraid of. *I don't play well with others. I always have to be the best at everything. No one will ever know the real me, and that is the way I like it.* All of these are example of fear-based thoughts that at one point may have kept that person safe, but now, just cause worry, isolation, and a barrier to a values-filled life.

For others, compartmentalizing your thoughts from who you are is extremely easy in theory, but a difficult task to carry out. We are going to start the process of separating who we are from what we think and giving each their own space.

When we find ourselves in the throes of anxiety, we are letting every thought that comes through our head give us a jolt of pressure, of heat, of sickness. I used to experience a fireball pit in my stomach searing its way through my existence during the bad times. It was dreadful. These feelings often do not motivate us to take action on anything we are worried about, especially since we are distracted by other worries. The thought of never being able to do it perfectly or never getting it done at all can be overpowering.

Anxiety is the reason we wait until hard deadlines are directly ahead. Procrastination is actually a symptom of anxiety, because anxiety is the process of worrying about something rather than just doing it. Intrinsically, we cannot seem to find our flow or motivation in a particular task with all those worry thoughts flying around. These little Joule Thieves have stolen our energy and focus and left us exhausted without anything to show for it.

Hopefully in the previous chapter you started to visualize yourself in a place where you have taken back control from these thoughts and can live your best life. We will learn here to grab one thought at a time, label it, and place it where it belongs. This chapter will dive into how to compartmentalize your thoughts, learn to prioritize tasks, and leave yourself time and energy to enjoy your life. Much like the energy budgeting we did earlier, this is putting thoughts and ideas into places and being aware of not only how much we are going to put into them (energy wise) but when. Our brain can relax knowing there is a time and place for each thing. As we feel more confident in our abilities to compartmentalize and prioritize, we can start applying this to more areas of stress in our lives.

EXCELLENT DAY PLANNER

Let me introduce you to the Excellent Day Planner. The first time I used one was in my PhD program. I had just finished my third semester of full-time classes, coupled with my research and clinical responsibilities, being a mom, and trying to keep myself healthy. I found myself in the heat of a North Carolina summer with no schedule and six comprehensive exams looming at the end of the summer. I also had my entire dissertation lurking in my thoughts, causing some fear-based thinking of *Will I ever finish it?*, or more accurately, *Will I even start it?* For the first time, no one was there to tell me when to be where, and I had to organize studying for all six exams, worries about dissertation, responsibilities of being a single mom to two young boys, self-care, caffeination, and eating time. I wandered into the neighboring PhD office to see if my friend Q'Nesha was at her cubby, and hopefully lament to her, a fellow student in the same point of the program as me. I found my saving grace. Instead of lamenting, she took one look at my face and handed me a copy of her day planner. She came up with the first version of this page and I have only expanded on it slightly since them. This helped me take all those anxious thoughts and find a place for them. I used to even schedule time to be anxious, which I soon needed less and less. Often, I'd schedule some sort of physical activity after my worry time to work off that cortisol! The first part of the activity will be identifying fear-based thoughts as actionable or irrelevant, and we will look at a list of common irrational thought patterns to help you decide where that thought belongs. Then we will take our actionable tasks and find a spot for them on the Excellent Day Planner.

As I got better at chunking down my worries and focusing on one thing at a time, I started to apply this to other areas of my life. One major worry many people have is related to finances. I started to open different bank accounts and label them different things to help me stay on top of spending. I have a business and personal one, of course, and then I have a Vacation Account, a Presents Account for Christmas or birthdays, a House Account, and so on. Some may be on the empty side, but if I have one particular goal, I do make an effort to create an account and work toward it. I chunk away at it. Another way I have embraced this is in food prep. I will find a particular food I want to eat and find ways to incorporate it throughout the week. Occasionally I get my kids on board, but often they have their own ideas on what they want to eat and can make it with minimal help. The less I must utilize energies working on these areas, the more I can put into my values. I don't think I would have ever finished this book without compartmentalizing and prioritizing my time and energy! In the appendix you will find a worksheet to practice taking a task and chunking it down.

PLANNED WORRY TIME

Yes, you read it right. Those little Joule Thieves? Well they tend to be quiet if you feed them a little bit. Tell them when their nap time is and give them a play time. As we work on compartmentalizing, set some time aside for these worries weekly, daily if you need to.

Use the Excellent Day Planner Handout to help with the activities in this chapter or create your own! There are resources online that may guide you as well.

The third activity in this chapter, the Mindset Shift, is an idea that grew from a YouTube video called "Leaves on a Stream." An intern who worked with me introduced me to this video and I love having it on as I organize my thoughts. This activity helps us slow down and take time to observe our thoughts and I have found it to be helpful to do this before working on compartmentalizing, so in this chapter the mindset shifting activity comes first!

ACTIVITY ONE:
COMPARTMENTALIZING YOUR THOUGHTS:
LEAVES ON A STREAM

Materials:

- Your mind and a quiet place

- Streaming device if you decide to use the YouTube video

1. As we've started to learn, anxiety is the great talent of worrying about all things at once. Often as we start to put words and labels on these worries, they become manageable. Each of our thoughts in this exercise gets our undivided attention as it floats in, and then it floats out and we wait for the next one, giving us an ability to separate these thoughts and deal with one thing as a time.

2. Read these directions or follow along with the audio. Find a quiet place where you will not be interrupted for five minutes. Close your eyes and get in touch with your breath. After a few long deep breaths, start this activity.

    Wait for a thought to pop in your head: *Don't forget to write down milk on the grocery list. Remember to text your sister. How much chocolate cake did I eat last night?*

    Imagine as you inhale that your thought expands in words across your mind. Hold your breath for a count, then as you exhale, imagine that thought slowly become particles of the words that form it, little silver particles that fall neatly into the area on your mind's planner page they belong. Is there a worries section box?

A social connections box? Family? Work? House? Imagine it falling neatly into that box as you inhale, wait a beat, and exhale.

Next thought, next breath. Just keep moving on. Each thought has its own place, and as they disperse into particles they are neatly put in their box because you are in control.

You have the power to decide which box you open and when.

ACTIVITY TWO:
UNPACK YOUR BRAIN

Materials:

- Laptop or writing pad and writing utensil

1. The first activity in this chapter has helped you connect to your thoughts and separate them from a giant ball of knotted strings to one string of thought at a time. Now we're going to take those individual strings and put them all where they belong.

2. To start this activity, open a Word document or a blank piece of paper. Give yourself five minutes to allow all the random stuff that floated down the stream or came to you in the last activity to flow out onto the paper. As a client once told me, your brain is for creativity and a notebook is for memory–anything you are trying to hold on to, just let it sit in this open document. No matter how disorganized it looks, it doesn't matter since no one else will see this but you. You are allowed to just let it flow. Sometimes it means dumping the things that are stopping your flow.

3. Write down how you feel after your brain dump. Relief? Disgust? Anywhere in between? Think about how your body feels. If your body feels lighter in any way, than the brain dump has done its job and you are ready to start prioritizing and compartmentalizing. As more rubbish gets in the way of your brain, remember the observation of thought activity. Let that leaf float its way down the stream, and if it tries to come back,

you brain dump it into that open document or notebook. No room for that in our Excellent Day.

4. Change your internal dialogue for the day. Look at the Excellent Day Planner Page included in this chapter.

    The top says: Goal of the Day. Think broadly about what you want that goal to be. Is it something concrete like finishing a task? Is it reminding yourself of something more existential like attitude is everything? Is it remembering funny things about your dad who has passed and writing them down during the day? This is really about you and what you want to drive you throughout the day, and where you'd like to reroute your extra energy for the day. Write it in your spot on the daily planner sheet.

    The next activity will guide you through deciding what tasks belong on the sheet, and what other times you need to chunk off for yourself.

ACTIVITY THREE:
PRIORITIZING WITH THE EXCELLENT DAY PLANNER:
COMMENCE CONTROL OF YOUR DAY

Materials:

- Excellent Day Planner Pages

- Writing utensil or laptop

1. Time to compartmentalize and prioritize. After your brain dumping exercise, you are now free to move about the brain. You can *choose* what you are going to focus on today and this week. Look at the daily planner. You may need to have a week's worth of daily planner pages out, or you may be better off just doing one day at a time. You decide what is right for you. Look at the goal of the day you have written. Be mindful of it as you go about this activity.

2. Before chunking down your time on the planner, think about the thoughts that were swirling around before that are now living on a paper and not in your mind. What tasks are relevant to your day and week? What were some worries that you can start to turn into actionable goals and chunk down some time to accomplish? Make a list of the time chunks you will need to have in each day. Include non-working days if those are tough days for to get through, or don't include them—decide for yourself what you need.

3. Start planning your time. Chunk off bits of time to get things done. If you think something will take you six hours, decide whether you want to chunk off six hours for it on Monday, or one hour per day for Monday through Saturday. Remember to put in at least fifteen-minute breaks throughout your day to detox your brain and rest it, uncoil it, and give it a chance not to produce cortisol or hyper focus. This is a test run. You may find that you need longer or shorter work periods, or longer or shorter breaks. It will take you a good few weeks of planning to get into the swing of your own rhythm and start organizing your tasks, worries, and breaks in a way that works best for you.

Things you may want to include on your schedule:

• Work directed Tasks (Break these down as small as possible)

• Gym time

• Food prep time

• Social media scrolling or updating

• Eating time

• Checking email

• Down time (to do absolutely nothing!)

• Check in time (Calling parents, partner, kids, friends)

• Caffeination and socialization (Hydration if you're not into the caffeine)

• Worry time (dedicated time to just identify what you're worrying about)

• Planner writing time (you need some time to make your daily planner!!)

Break your tasks into achievable chunks by breaking them into smaller pieces. Use the *What Am I Doing* section to chunk down your time.

Here's an example: If you are worried about writing a paper, chunk it down each day until it is due. From 8:15 a.m. to 8:45, work on inputting references and formatting. From 9 to 10:15, organize what is already written and check for grammar. From 10:30 to 11 write new material. Take a break at 11 a.m. for lunch and call your bud. The next day from 8:15-8:45 read it through. From 11-12 edit and give it the once over. Write down a reminder to submit the finished product before the due date.

There are a few examples of daily planner pages to give you some other ideas as well. The main goal is to chunk things you are worrying about down into achievable goals, and to put them on your planner in terms of priority. If something is due on Tuesday, make time for it on Monday and put something else on the back burner. You have a spot on the Excellent Day Planner page to write your top three energy priorities of the day as a friendly reminder going about your day. If the paper is due before your presentation in two weeks, make sure you are putting more energy into the paper by chunking more time for it than the presentation. That goes at the top of your energy priority list.

4. Don't forget self-care! In addition to scheduling chunks of your day for down time, the bottom gives you a space to check off water and meal consumption, as well as exercise. You might be pretty regimented with that stuff and not need that area, so don't stress. Use it if you need to.

5. There are a few other sections to use as you desire. There is a Daily Inspiration section you can use to write your values words, an affirmation, or anything that helps you stay on track

throughout the day. There is Good Things of Today section to note your accomplishments (and not focus on your worries). And there is a spot to finish this statement: "Today I aligned my energy with my values by_____." Try to find time to think about how you will fill out this statement at the end of each day. The more concrete you are with your words, the more you control your thoughts!

6. At the end of the week, take a few minutes to think about what worked and what did needs tweaking. What are three things you can do to streamline the process and keep your tank full all week long? Start working on next week's planner pages before the week begins.

CHAPTER SIX

BIG PICTURE GOAL SETTING

How many times have you heard someone say, "I work better under pressure" or "I need a deadline." Have you said those things yourself? We create distress to trick our brain to complete an activity to avoid distress instead of to enjoy accomplishment.

In this day and age, there is so much pressure put on us from every angle: Peers, bosses, teachers, parents, wives, girlfriends, husbands, boyfriends. Then there's social media, the news, advertisements, all setting ideals for us that are realistically unattainable. There's financial pressure from living in a society where two incomes can barely get you by. There's merit-based pressure of having to compare your success with the success of others. There's relationship-based pressure from others to meet their expectations. And then with anxiety, we go ahead and pile more pressure on ourselves. That seems healthy! It's no wonder we have learned that we need pressure to complete anything. We've been conditioned to focus on the completion of tasks and not on the joy of the process–where does that task lead us?

When we zoom out, we can reset our perspective on what we are worrying about. Some questions to explore in the big picture are:

- How do this affect my life right now in this moment?

- Is there any relevant action that can be taken in the moment?

- Is there a decision I am avoiding or adding pressure to?

• Is the pressure necessary in the moment?

Zooming out is taking each worry into a perspective–a broader perspective than the rabbit hole it leads you down. I like the imagery of opening a door versus peering through the peephole. The latter distorts what you are seeing and makes it larger than life. You know how big someone's nose looks when you stare through that thing! That's what hyper focusing on our worries does. When we zoom out, we are opening the door and not only broadening our perspective but seeing it more realistically.

PERCEIVED PRESSURE

Now that we've broken tasks and worries down into small achievable pieces, we are going to focus on differentiating between real pressure and what I call "perceived pressure." That is the pressure we put on ourselves, because of expectations or standards we hold for ourselves, for those around us, and for our environment/ reality. When we have not compartmentalized and broken down our worries, we often cannot fully understand determine what expectations we have that are not being met. Now that we've decluttered, we can be clear about what expectations and goals we hold for ourselves, and what is within our control on the way to reaching them. Perceived pressure is feeling like you must be the best, the first, the funniest, the most in-control, without any real consequence for that achievement in the big picture.

One aspect of human existence rife with perceived pressures are romantic relationships. Especially in the dating phase. I work with many clients who are unhappy or unfulfilled because they feel like they need to find love, and that their life cannot be complete without it. Let's look at an example of perceived pressure and separate that from real pressures and responsibilities.

A client named Janet came to see me due to anxiety that had cropped up in her graduate program studies. Although that was the stressor she presented, every session Janet would inevitably discuss the "should I/should I nots" of getting back together with an ex-lover, Simon. Worrying about it was causing her to abandon her studies, isolate from friends, and even spends hours on the internet researching relationship advice (as well as take up a good portion of her counseling sessions). She was so *zoomed in* and putting so much pressure on herself and this decision.

How many of us can relate with some part of Janet's story? What she was dealing with was a whole lot of perceived pressure—made up entirely by the Joule Thief that is anxiety.

When we zoomed out on the situation, we walked through the best-case scenario Janet could imagine as an outcome. Janet's best-case scenario was getting back together with Simon, and then either staying together in a healthier relationship or eventually breaking up with him knowing they had given it their best shot.

We went through what her worst-case scenario imaginable would be. In this scenario, Janet gets back together with Simon, only to be dumped in public and be embarrassed in front of all her friends. We discussed which pieces of this scenario she was hyper focused on or "zoomed in." She was worrying about a particular incident in the future where Simon purposefully embarrasses her. In reality, Simon had been a very supportive, non-confrontational person, so dumping her in front of all her friends at a big gathering would be unprecedented and out of character.

When we discussed where this particular scenario came from, she started to zoom out and realize it was her anxiety that had created this possible future scenario to avoid her getting hurt again. The ever-creative Joule Thief had played upon many insecurities Janet had, including seeming "wishy-washy" about getting back to together with Simon, social anxiety about big parties, along with the chance of being embarrassed and hurt by Simon. Some of these anxieties dated back to early childhood and healing from them became a focus of our work rather than her making a decision right now about her relationship.

Janet's anxiety had melted together to create a disastrous worst-case scenario that was highly unlikely. This was a creative design by Janet's Joule Thief to keep her from "taking a risk" and making a decision her brain perceived might hurt her. Remember, we may call anxiety a "thief" but as far as anxiety is concerned, it is protecting our hide from all the crazy things we think we can do without getting hurt!

How did perceived pressure play into Janet's situation? She put so much pressure on making the right decision right now and did not think about how in the larger picture, making that decision was not going to change everything or cause her as much distress as she was imagining. And in reality, she did not have to know what was going to happen in the relationship. Trying to guess what the outcome would be had stolen her energy away from enjoying time now with Simon. She wasn't spending much time listening or accurately reading input from him and instead was letting her anxiety steal away her focus and create scenarios that were both unlikely to occur and out of her control. If the only way she could control them was to just not be with Simon, what kind of a decision would that be? What kind of life is built around no risk?

TWENTY - SEVEN MILES TO EMPTY

Driving along, that "ding" signals I'm low on gas.
Well in my old Ford, it would tell me how many miles
I had left until it was empty. It started at fifty, then it would ding
again at forty. Then for some reason it would ding again
at twenty-seven, not thirty.

And it was that number, that finite,
specific number twenty-seven that finally got me to stop
what I was doing, pull into a gas station,
and get some gas before I was floundering stranded on I-264?
or worse, waiting for help to come.

One day while waiting for an eternally slow gas pump to rejuvenate
my car and bring my back to independence,
I had a dynamic realization.
I don't just wait until I'm twenty-seven miles to empty for my car.
I do it in EVERYTHING.

I need a deadline looming over me like the Gloom Man from my
childhood nightmares until I finally sit down
and do something to relieve the pit in my stomach.
Even years of working through these and practicing what this
chapter is about - differentiating between real stressors and
perceived pressure. If I been able to prioritize and assign
a time/deadline for getting gas,
it would not become a stressor or cause anxiety.

Janet realized that making the wrong decision was a concept she'd made up in her mind without her consent. She was not living her value-filled life due to trying to control a future her anxiety had dreamed up. The Joule Thief was rich while Janet was struggling to keep her grades, relationships, and sanity.

In this chapter you will look at what perceived pressure you put on external events and relationships in your life, and work toward identifying what your internal script is trying to protect you from.

Often there are a few questions you can ask yourself to decide if the pressure you feel from a situation is intrinsic or extrinsic.

1. Is someone else affected by this decision more than me?

2. Am I putting my values onto that person?

3. Am I letting that person's (or group of people, even up to society) values make this decision for me?

So let's work on separating pressure into some different categories. We have real stressors—bills, jobs, families—that we have to factor into our energy spending. Then we have the perceived pressures we create for ourselves. Trying to please everyone. Trying to be the "best (fill in the blank) possible." Trying to be your fittest/thinnest/healthiest ever. Sometimes this goes over into perfectionism—having to do everything just right and then criticizing ourselves even when we gave our best.

Often when we think about perceived pressure, the word "should" is involved. We have a story we tell ourselves to every external event that occurs in our lives. If someone looks at us sideways, we might say:

I should not dress like such a slob. I should lose weight. I should smile more.

If we open a credit card statement:

I should be more careful with my money. I should have this paid off by now. I should be smarter than this.

If our kid is misbehaving in public:

I should be a better parent. I should have taught him how to act. I should not have to deal with this.

If we are on a date and the other person sends a text message:

I should not have come; they're not even interested in me. I should not try to meet people; they just talk bad about me.

I think you can think up various scenarios where these should statements come up for you.

Many people who come to me have rested their version of success on finding the right partner. Or the right job. Or the right amount of success. Can you relate in any way?

In the future, with that partner/job/success, you are allowed to relax, to be happy, and to feel fulfilled. That one thing can extend your happiness. With a partner, it will help feel like there is a shared history as you grow old, and they can be pleasurable to be around mentally, physically, and emotionally. With the job, you can enjoy your free time because you now know you've reached the pinnacle of success at work.

But what about right now? You are putting a limit on how happy, relaxed, and fulfilled you feel. This is what perceived pressure does—it limits our happiness in the moment. The following exercises will help you see where your energy goes and put reminders in place of your energy goals.

In the first activity we are going to" zoom in to zoom out". We will pick one situation and discover what narrative goes off in your brain.

We're going to look at the story you tell yourself in specific situations and find what your theme is.

Our story is often the foundation of how we describe every event that occurs in our lives and is what causes our anxiety/issues/problems, not the event or circumstance we see as the cause.

ACTIVITY ONE:
EVENT MAPPING:
THE ART OF THOUGHTFUL RESPONSE

Materials:

- Writing platform and utensil, be as creative as you'd like

This exercise will help you figure out how your perception of external events influences your reactions.

1. Think of an example of something that caused you distress in the last week. An external event like finding out you have a deadline for school or work you forgot about, or bumping into your ex at the post office, or the fact that it is raining out on a day you wanted to have a picnic. It doesn't matter how big or small the occurrence; If it caused you distress, it counts. I'll show you a picture of what this looks like when we write it out in the example below. My example external event is receiving a text message from your boss asking where the materials are, he asked you to send him today. Choose your event and make a circle around the event like this. Leave room for that Stop sign but we'll come back to it soon.

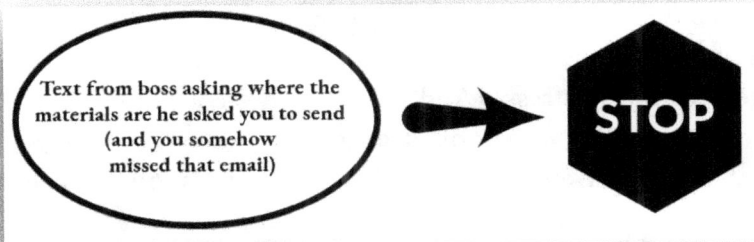

2. Write down the reaction that you had to the event. Make one bubble for your physical reaction, another one for your emotional.

3. Make a bubble for your action - How did you react in the moment to this event?

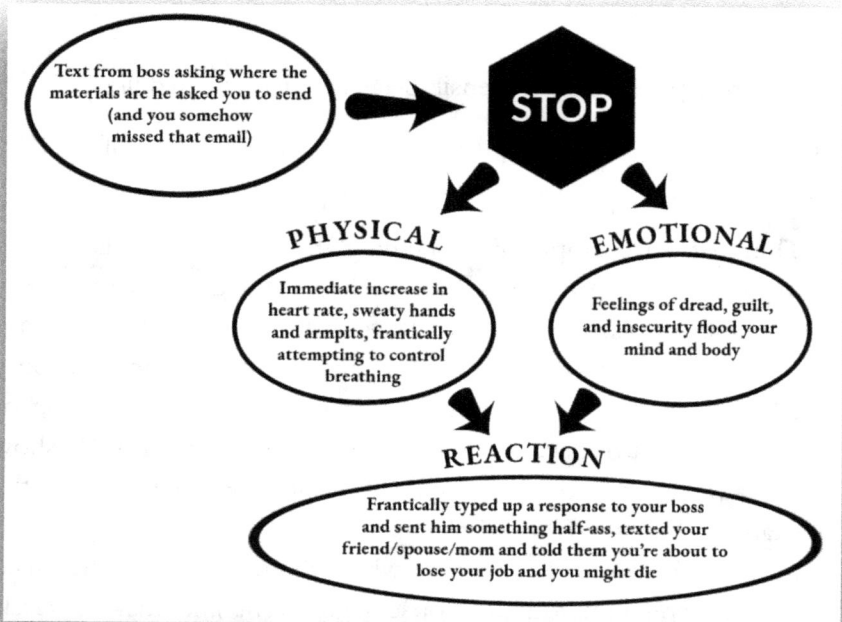

4. What are the long-term consequences of these actions? For mine, there is the physical risk of high blood pressure, coronary issues, IBS, and a host of other ailments with this kind of a response to stress. And relationally, connections become unhealthy. This can look like constant worrying and judging, jealousy, passive aggressive behaviors, or isolation. Your anxiety continues to be in control of your reactions.

REACTION

Frantically typed up a response to your boss and sent him something half-ass, texted your friend/spouse/mom and told them you're about to lose your job and you might die

↓

LONG TERM STRESS CONSEQUENCES

High blood pressure, coronary issues, IBS, and a host of other ailments

Withdrawal, isolation, jealousy, insecurity, disconnection

Loss of jobs, relationships, self-esteem, and self-regulation

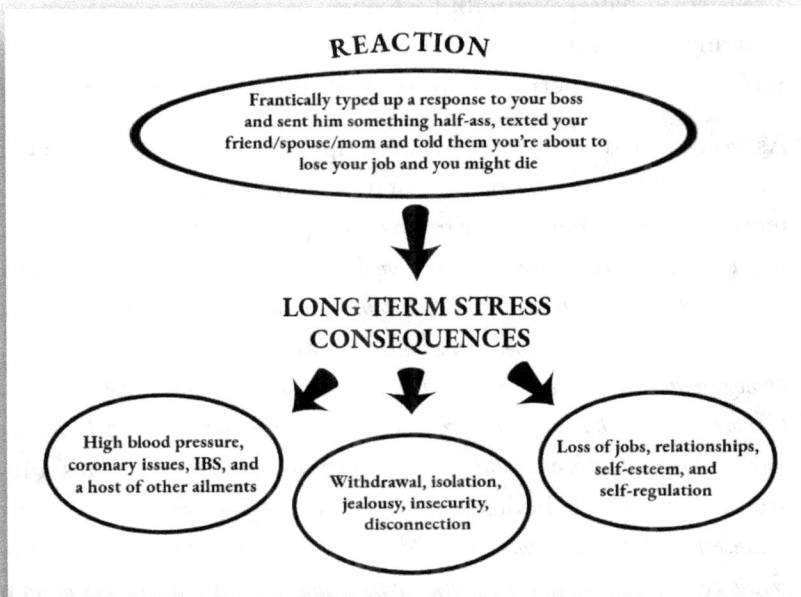

5. Now go back to the stop sign. What happened there? Are there other ways you could have responded to this event to create different short term and long-term consequences? Yes of course. So, here's how we get there.

We start to recognize the story we tell ourselves whenever an external event occurs. In this example, that story or script is what dictates the course of our reactions. When the email from the boss is read, the very first that happened is a script was called up to make sense of the situation. In this example, that script might have been, *I'm so dumb, why do I always let worrying about other things get in the way of remembering deadline. My boss is going to think I'm the stupidest person on the planet and fire me immediately* or some variation. The instant response *to* that script (not to the external event) is to fire off a half-ass attempt at the material he asked for and freaking out to all those close to you that you might lose your job—and sort of perpetuating your script in the first place, right?

As you start to recognize what scripts start running the second you get fired up, you can start using your superpowers to recognize and then re-write that script in a more realistic and more empowering manner. *Hmm. I am going to back in my emails and make sure that the boss did indeed send me an email asking for this, and then figure out where the communication was lost along the way. I will apologize to him and explain where the communication was dropped and tell him when I can have the materials to him by, keeping in mind I still want them to be my best work and not something half-ass.* Maybe that's a high arching script. Maybe it's something like, *I feel like I might freak out because I can't believe I missed this deadline, but I KNOW that I am a good employee, my boss values my work or he would not have asked me to do this in the first place, and I can find a solution to this problem if I give myself a minute to process.* Now, your body response is going to be calmer, maybe a slight fluttering of the heart and a little extra sweat on your palms, but nowhere near where you worked yourself up before. Your response will be well thought out and your boss will see you keep a cool head under pressure. Your texts to loved ones won't be distraught and dramatic, but even keeled. The long-term consequences are the opposite of everything we listed before—lower blood pressure, better connections, higher self-esteem, and maintenance of long-term relationships.

6. Practice this first with something that happened in the past. The more you practice rewriting your scripts, the more you will be able to handle these situations in the moment. Practice the art of thoughtful response rather than reactive negative behaviors.

ACTIVITY TWO:
A POCKET FULL OF SUNSHINE

Materials:

- Post-its

- Writing utensil

This is an exercise that serves as a helpful reminder for re-writing your script.

1. Think of a mental cue to remember your thoughtful response script—maybe the word is a general cue, like "empowerment" or "positivity." Maybe it's someone's name that brings to mind a role model for how to act. Or just a phrase like "Knowing I can handle what comes my way" or "Adaptable and Kind." Write this note on your first Post-it. Place it in your right pocket or somewhere close to you on the right.

2. Now think of a word that you want to avoid—something that has to do with your negative script, or even a person you may NOT want to react like. It could be "fear" or "self-conscious" or "negative" or it could be something like, "Worthless employee of the month" or "I'm never good enough." Write that on your second Post-it. Put that in your left pocket or somewhere close on that side of you.

3. Every time you remember that day, reach toward the Post-it on your right and take it out and read it. Remember that this is where you want to go every time a situation presents itself to you in life. Anytime you reach and find yourself in contact with the

Post-it on the left, remember that thought pathway is something you will always carry with you, but you have the choice to put it back and reach to the right every time you cross its path.

Here's another visualization activity that helps with
Zooming OUT:
The sand dollar and the number five share symbolism.
The sand dollar has been referred to as the five-pointed star of the sea - a powerful totem of the necessary changes to move from dimension to the next. The sand dollars we see on the beach are dead sea creatures, that transform from living beings to collectible fragile coveted "beach money." Visualize yourself on the beach. Feel the sand under your toes, the tiny pieces of sea debris under your feet. The smell of sea teases your nostrils on the breeze. You feel the waves lap your feet, and you look down to see what they left behind for you. A half sand dollar is sticking out of the sand by your feet. You bend down to pick it up, and you immediately notice this former life form is more delicate than any shell you've picked up. You must carefully hold it, not wrapping your fingers too closely around it lest it break some more. Amazed at its fragile nature, you think of how many storms and waves this sand dollar has survived in the sea, only to land by your feet and by at the mercy of your hands. You must be gentle in your approach to the sand dollar, regardless of how many harsh environmental conditions it has been exposed to.
Much like you need to be to yourself in this process.

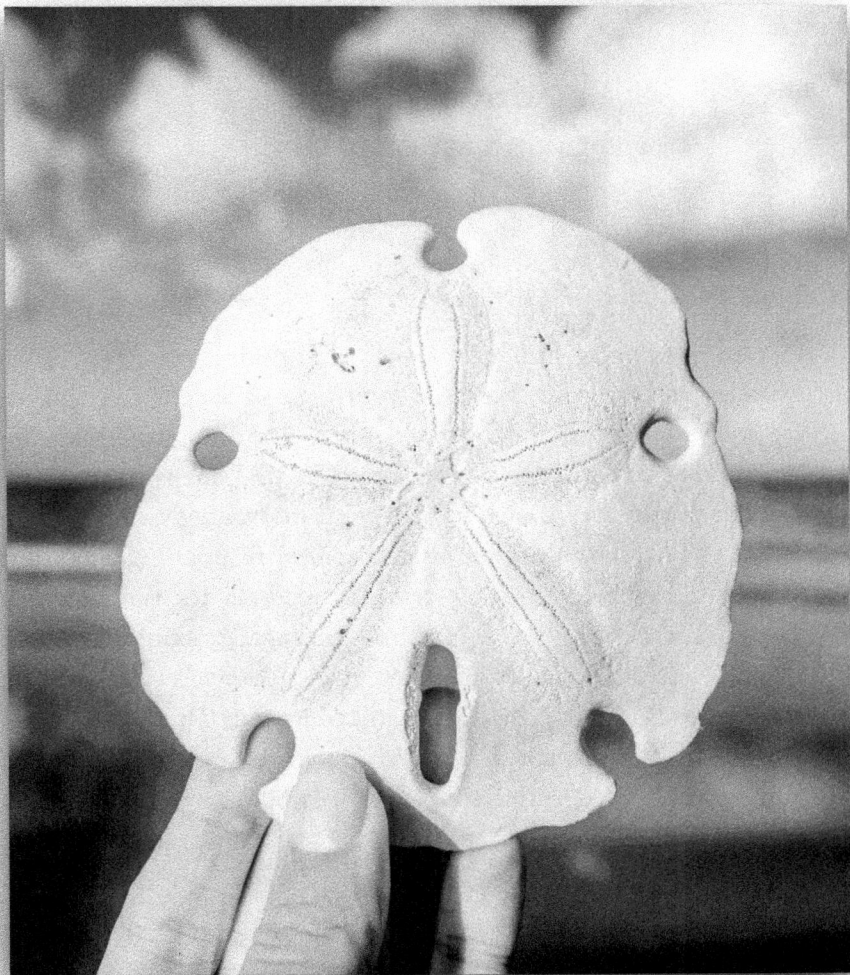

ACTIVITY THREE:
LIVING MY BEST LIFE

Materials:

- Just your brain

1. Picture a stressful situation. Feel your bodily response. What expression is on your face? Are your hands relaxed? Legs? What are you holding on to? Now, remember your thoughtful response script and how you want to respond to that stressful situation. Take back control of each part of your body slowly, one piece at a time. Visualize yourself in that situation, responding according to the thoughtful response script. Instead of focusing on that situation, imagine yourself in the present, walking down an avenue. Anything could come up at you as you walk–you've never been here. But you feel relaxed and prepared. This is the safest place you've ever walked because you've released the perceived pressure and the negative scripts you placed in your life, and you are now living from a place of thoughtful response. Walk down this avenue until you reach the end, where you can sit in a comfortable, quiet spot and rest as long as you like. You are ready now, for whatever comes your way.

CHAPTER SEVEN

WRITING IT ALL DOWN

In Pursuit of The Whole Sand Dollar was conceived through my journaling. I've never had a more meaningful breakthrough than that one on the shore, where I recognized how I was spending my energy. It has changed every single thing about my work moving forward. At that point I saw with clarity how much energy I was spending on people, places, and ideals that didn't align with my personal values. The idea of the broken sand dollar has repaired me in more ways than I can describe.

Sometimes we can find these meaningful breakthroughs in other ways of expression. I hope that you discover an outlet for your creativity, whether it's writing, artwork, or otherwise, that helps you realign your energy to live a values-filled life as well. Here we focus on writing, but you can always substitute the activity for using the prompts in art, body work, yoga, or any sort of expressive activity you choose. The research in writing and journaling is extensive and I focus on that here, but you can do what speaks to you.

So how much can writing really help? For centuries, writing has been used as a source of healing. The act of writing gives us the chance to put words to our feelings as well as grow personally in terms of self-expression and self-awareness and understanding. It also gives us the experience of feeling heard or understood by others. This can decrease feelings of isolation and increase our resiliency in times of stress. Research shows that writing fifteen to thirty minutes a day, three days a week can significantly reduce stress and offer other cathartic benefits.[6]

But if we have these anxieties, we sometimes can't even put a name to, how do we write about it?

Just sit and start writing.

I often suggest this as the first step. Give yourself even five minutes of nonstop "pen to page" time to start and just see what comes out. Increase this time as much as you can, up to thirty minutes.

Our most common—misunderstandings with communications cause us anxiety and excessive worry (Example: *My boss just called me in his office, I must be getting fired!*) and we don't even realize why. Once we can find the words to convey what we fear in this situation, we can then start working on mindset interventions that will help us settle our minds and gain back control.

The field of neuro-counseling is expanding rapidly, which is very exciting for people like me who specialize in helping get your brain's shenanigans back under your control. We now know which parts of the brain activate in anxious states, depressive states, trauma states, and so much more. One thing that's been found is that the words used to describe worries, situations, and relationships literally rewire our brain for us. I hate mice, and I could tell you some reasons why —though I prefer not to—but I can deal with seeing them or the telltale signs of them now that I think of them as baby elephant friends. It has something to do with the part of my brain that is hardwired for empathy and its relationship to how elephants feel about how I treat mice rather than how I feel about mice in general. I have rewired my brain through a story I wrote in journaling one day to not be so oversensitive to the sensory or verbal input associated with seeing a mouse. All by changing the story I tell myself.

Those who are gifted with words can access their unconscious behaviors and thoughts in a more tangible form. Those who are not, become more adept at putting words to obscure what ifs. It's as if they are taking back some control from the thought that was floating which has now been caught concretely on paper.

In Volume 13 (2018) of the *Journal of Creativity in Mental Health*, researchers Gladding and Wallace have a great article that list examples of writing exercises that can help with mental health. I have used many of these successfully with clients. Their research discusses the link between writing and dealing with our emotions and worries.

ACTIVITY ONE:
BRAIN DUMP 101
(FIVE MINUTES OF FREE WRITING)

Materials:

- Paper

- A writing implement

1. Research supports the idea that writing and reading your own handwriting activates your brain more intently than reading something you typed on an electronic device. So unless there is a physical reason to avoid the pen/paper route, let's just humor research for today and try it. Make sure you have at least ten minutes free for this first attempt at therapeutic writing. As soon as your timer goes off, start writing about anything. This one is prompt free. Once you get in the flow, you will feel the words start jumping onto the page. If you don't, start by writing one word over and over until other words come. The point is to allow your brain to purge (or "dump") all the miscellaneous content taking up space and allow it to access the real problems. It's like pulling a few pieces of hair out of your shower drain when you know you really need to take the cover off and deep clean it with chemicals. That's what we're about to do: Commence a deep clean.

2. Try to do this exercise at least three times this week. You do not have to reread your material or keep it for any future use (but you can if you'd like). This is strictly to purge our brain of any unnecessary surface material and get down to the core of what we want to focus on, whether it be problems or solutions. See if

you can incorporate this activity into your life over the next month and move up to thirty-minute sessions at least once a week. This will really keep you fresh and primed to deal with whatever comes your way, especially if you are continuing to do the other exercises suggested in the book. Think about it as taking out the trash. You don't want to leave that piling up each week!

ACTIVITY TWO:
PROMPT WRITING

Materials:

- A writing implement

- Paper

- A prompt

1. Here's where you choose your own adventure. Either choose a prompt below or make up your own. Better yet, write each prompt down on a piece of paper and fold them up, placing them all in an envelope. Other the course of the few weeks, each time you sit down to write, choose a new paper out of the envelope before you start. That way you don't have any time to stress about the prompt or what you are going to write. It just flows.

Prompt examples:

- What is something you are continually working on within yourself?

- What would you do if you loved yourself unconditionally?

- Talk about what is *enough* for you.

- Write about a time when work felt real to you, necessary, and satisfying (paid or unpaid, professional or domestic, physical or mental).

- Write the words you need to hear right now.

These prompts speak to common core beliefs that fuel our anxiety, and our common stressors. Or look for some that really speak to you. Check out the Additional resources on page 127 for more ideas.

2. Go back and briefly look over what you've written. Can you sum up in one sentence what your biggest takeaway is from that writing? Can you make it into a goal?

ACTIVITY THREE:
A LETTER TO MY FORMER PRESENT SELF

Materials:

- A writing implement

- Paper

1. Start with a fresh piece of paper. Set up the top as if you were writing a letter to yourself at your present address. Date it five years in the future. Before you write anything else, recall your perfect day from Chapter Four. Your future self is living this version of your life every day. Close your eyes and remember what that looks like, what that feels like, smells like, sounds like. Put yourself there.

2. Write a letter to yourself. This letter is from your future self to your present self. This future self has reached all the goals you set out at the beginning of this book, and perhaps even earlier than that. Then, put pen to paper and start writing. Let your present self know what-you to help get you to where you are now. Let yourself know what it feels like to live that life. Let yourself know the impact it has had on others in your life. Let yourself know what you can do today to start moving toward that life.

These activities can be repeated as needed. Journaling as a lifelong habit can redirect negative thoughts and feelings on a regular basis, helping you live a healthier life day to day. Although the readings and exercises in this book are designed to be completed in a few months, hopefully some of the activities, become a permanent part of your life. These daily habits are what create the greatest change in our life and help us become that best version of ourselves.

CHAPTER EIGHT

IF YOU CAN'T GET CLOSURE, MAKE CLOSURE

We've worked hard together over the last several chapters. We have separated what we care about from what steals our energy. We've learned to break down stressors into achievable chunks, and how to work hard toward our goals. We've worked at focusing on our minds on what we really care about. We have replaced some of our fear-based thoughts with empowered ones. We have brain dumped our negativity and worry and cleansed our brain for new ideas and chapters to come. After all of that, now we're ready to work on a little closure.

One place we often look for closure is in relationships. Whether it's a fight with a loved one, or a disagreement with a boss or coworker, or the breaking up with a romantic partner, all of us have in some way searched for the reasoning behind why things happened. Like our childhood fables with morals at the end, we feel we need to succinctly put into words what we've learned and the why of it all before we can move on. Sometimes without this, we feel broken. When I am working through closure, I give myself one sentence to wrap the situation in my head. When it comes to relationships, I can share it with others, but oftentimes it is just for me.

Without the closure we seek from the other person, we allow ourselves to feel the burn of the cut and then was ask, what's our healthiest choice?

Find our own way to close the wound.

113

Re-read the title of this chapter. We're going to go through how to do that externally within the situation to alleviate that stuck circuitry in our brain seeking closure from others. Then we're going to "disengage, turn the page, and move to the next stage. "

One of the wisest, kindest professors (and people) I ever had the pleasure to know helped me find this solution and catchy phrase. I was a little late and apparently frazzled-seeming when I showed up at his office one day for a meeting. We were working on the stats for my dissertation, but it was more than that overwhelming feat. He asked me what was going on, so I told him—I had a "friend" I had realized was very toxic for me. I had tried the "friend breakup," tried talking about why I didn't have time right now to pursue the kind of friendship they wanted. But in the 14-minute drive to school from my house, she had sent me seventy-two text messages. Seventy-two. "That's quite a bit of messages," my professor said when I told him. I asked if he had any advice what to say to her. "Disengage. Do not say another thing."

In toxic relationships, the best we can do is not give them any ammo. Even a quick yes or no answer can be enough to spur them on again. I couldn't believe that was his advice. It was so simple, and not very person-centered to me. But then I realized it was person-centered. To me. In order for this to be healthy for me, I had to disengage. Even though I only sent about four texts for the seventy-two, that was four too many. So, I put the phone away and we started working.

I noticed as we were moving through the stats, instead of turning the page in my notebook to take more notes, I was using the same page, writing in the margins, making arrows to try and make sense the scribble. I was frustrated with myself. *Why don't I just turn the page?*

Grrr. Again, he stopped and looked at me. He said, "Disengage, turn the page." This seems to be a common theme.

Out of someone else's mouth I may not have paid attention, but this phrase has changed the way I interact with the world. Without that simple phrasing, I would be stuck in so many of these situations.

I find myself not only stopping the expenditure of energy on toxic people, but I have SO MUCH more energy for those that I love. These toxic people and relationship are some of the most common Joule Thieves we have. They suck our energy on a daily basis, and often we feel there is no way out. Or they end things with us in a way that leaves us searching for an answer to "what did I do wrong" when really the relationship itself was all wrong for you in the first place.

But how does one turn the page and move to the next stage? I've broken this down for you as well.

There are other areas in our life where we would like closure and cannot always achieve it by relying on the other person. This causes our anxiety to kick in big time, because our brain responds to any social threat like loss of an important relationship as a survival threat that threatens our safety.

I am offering a solution to your brain's desire for closure. If we give it an answer with finality to it, we can then close that chapter and move forward.

So, activity one is a way to communicate your piece, and regardless of whether or not you get a response, know that you communicated without any sort of word vomit or things to regret later. And that is closure–communicating your piece.

ACTIVITY ONE:

THE ABC'S OF GETTING CLOSURE:

UNDERSTAND YOUR OWN POINT OF VIEW

Materials:

- Writing materials

1. I am looking at a dry erase board right now. I like to have my options editable. But what we are going to do in this activity can be done with just a pen and paper or even a voice recorder. We're going to break your communication for closure down into three simple pieces:

   A. What you are looking for (action-oriented)

   B. What is confusing you or preventing closure (behavior)

   C. Where you'd like to leave it with the other person or situation, regardless of their intention (conclusion)

Choose a situation where you would like some closure. It can be a relationship, a financial situation, a worry about the future, a regret from the past- you choose.

Look at the three questions above, and start to create a statement that covers A. What action you are looking for to seek closure, B. What is preventing that closure for you, and C. Where you would like to leave it- the conclusion. The dry erase board gives me the ability to change things as I go and put it in an order that makes the most sense. So, your closure statement may be in BCA format, or CBA, but it will have the three components, somewhere.

I'm going to walk you through a few examples.

When things get murky in relationship I like to look at it like this–I am never going to know exactly where that person is in this murkiness, but if I make my own place known, they have the chance to reciprocate.

We ask ourselves so many questions. *What did that mean when they did that? Why did they say, "good night" and not "good-night, baby? Is something wrong? How do I know how they feel/what to wear/where to go/ if I should text them or not?"*

Here's an example. Sally goes on a date with Taylor. She feels like it went well but isn't sure what Taylor thinks. Chances are the same though, right? But she hasn't heard back from Taylor. Sally sends a text that says "Great date "with a smiley face afterwards. It's now been eighteen hours after their date ended and the text was sent. Sally thinks to herself, "What could possibly have gone wrong? Did I say something that pissed Taylor off? Made Taylor unattracted to me?"

So instead of spending countless Energy Joules worrying about this, let's learn how to make closure for Sally (and for ourselves). Remember we can never control what other people do or say. We can only control our actions. So, we are going to tell Taylor: (a) what we would like/need/want, (b) why we're confused. And (c) what Taylor could do to alleviate situation.

Two examples of messages Sally could send is:

"Hey Taylor, I enjoyed our time together Tuesday and would love to hang out again! (A) I know you have a lot going on mid-week but haven't heard from you since our date and wanted to check in. (B) Let me know if you'd like to hang out again soon. (C) Take care."

OR

"Hey Taylor, I miss spending time together without all this shortness and weirdness that has started between us. I'm not sure what went wrong entirely, but I know we both miscommunicated and we haven't been able to get past it. (B. I'd love to talk and hear your point of view and help you understand where I'm coming from. (A) Let me know if we can move forward through this together and hang out tonight. If I don't hear from you, I'll understand you don't want to move forward at this point. (C)"

They don't have to necessarily stay in A-B-C order, as long as you communicate each piece directly.

Now, Sally may never hear from Taylor again. But her brain knows where she stands. She did not word vomit at them about all your feelings and insecurities. She didn't inundate them with text messages or emails. She simply stated her piece and then disengaged, moved on to the next stage. This gives Taylor some room to either move forward or persevere on the issue at hand. It also lets Taylor know where Sally stands without laying any blame or starting another fight. If Taylor reengages in a healthy way, which she has set him up to do, then her story can move on. If Taylor doesn't, she has a neat ending that stops the anxiety of "what ifs" in terms of communication. Once she has said her piece, Sally must turn the page and choose not to engage unless the outcomes are healthy and moving in a positive direction.

2. Play around with your statement until it sounds like your style of communication, gets the message across, and gives you a feeling of having said your piece (the only part in your control) and moving on. The situation may be ongoing, but you are clear where you stand and what you need to provide closure for yourself.

Welcome to the next stage.

ACTIVITY TWO:

JOURNAL PROMPT: CHAPTER NEW

Materials:

- Pen/Paper or computer

1. We're experts on the power of journaling, right? So, let's put it to use. This is where my sand dollar story began and evolved, and I hope you find your story of growth and freedom in here as well. Take back control from the Joule Thieves of your life and start living the Values-Filled Life you desire.

    Here's your prompt:

    Chapter New: What is in store on the next page?"

    Set a timer so you have at least ten minutes to work on this. Go over if you need to. But in detail, describe your next chapter. What is the goal? Who are the characters? What is the conflict being overcome? What lessons will be learned?

    When you are done writing, give yourself some space (at least fifteen minutes), and then come back to it.

ACTIVITY THREE:
LIVING YOUR NEW CHAPTER

1. Now that you wrote down your ideas on the next chapter for yourself, we are going to take some time to sit and visualize you living this Chapter New. Find a comfy place to sit, close your eyes, and bring yourself to the scene you've created in the new chapter. Think about your five senses and clue into this new environment- what do you see? What do you hear? What does the air feel like? What smells do you discover as you breathe in? What tastes do you experience? Spend as much time as you want in this new chapter, soaking it all in. As you open your eyes and breathe in a deep breath, remember, you are walking into this life now.

AFTERWORD

NOT MY SAND DOLLAR

I told you about the day that changed the way I live my life. Searching for the sand dollar on the beach. And the idea that the broken pieces were just as beautiful as that elusive whole sand dollar.

There was another important lesson the sand dollar shards taught me that day.

I put many of the pieces I collected in my hands that day back in the ocean. I selected a few that truly felt whole again when I held them in my hand. I placed them next to each other, noting how beautiful they looked on the sand next to each other.

There was something about them that inspired me and made me feel I was giving them energy by admiring their beauty and they were giving me some in return. Other pieces I had collected on my run were magnificent in their broken beauty, but I felt no connection when I held them, and I felt they didn't fit into the picture of the collected pieces. I felt no remorse as I put them back on the beach and walked back to the cottage with the pieces that had resonated with me.

I cannot collect all the broken pieces that show up to me. I have to listen very carefully to hear the ones that truly need me, the ones I can provide to and help them feel whole in their new form. The ones that give energy back to me through the process of healing, because they allow me to use my skills to help and heal.

I listen carefully to discern the difference between those whose needs are called to me, and those that will take too much of me because they do not truly need what I have to give. So there's enough of me left to be happy and whole. This is a muscle I'm trying to work on, to flex and make stronger and also to let rest and recover. Recovering may seem selfish on the surface. But doing so allows me to become a better version of myself. I am doing this by following the true calling the universe has set out for me and remembering that not all the broken pieces are mine to fix.

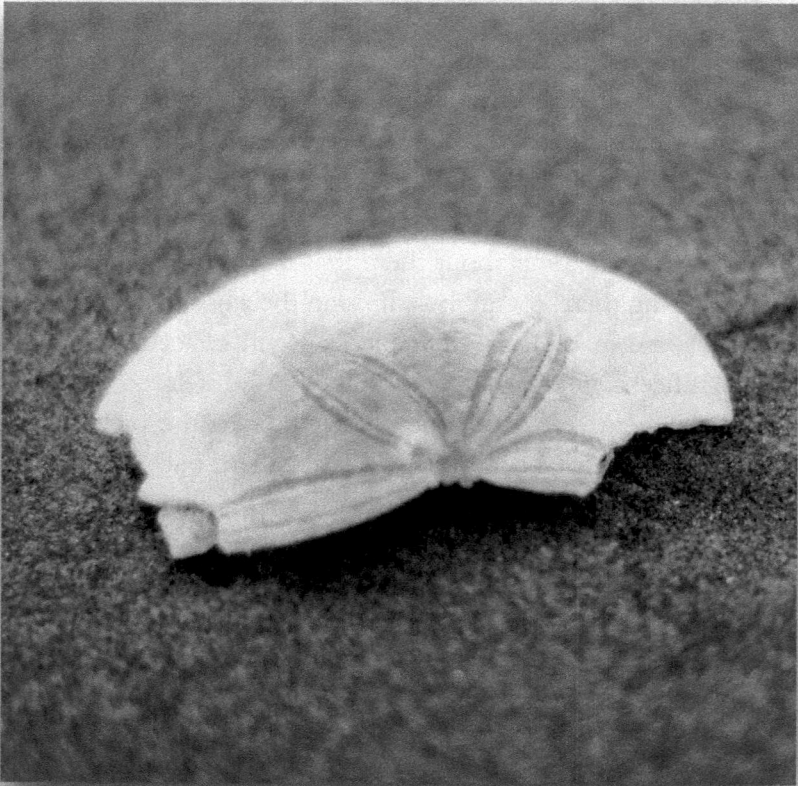

MY EXCELLENT DAY PLANNER

Date:

Focus of Today:

Daily Inspiration

Time	What Am I Doing?	🖋
6:00		✓ ✗ ↘
6:30		✓ ✗ ↘
7:00		✓ ✗ ↘
7:30		✓ ✗ ↘
8:00		✓ ✗ ↘
8:30		✓ ✗ ↘
9:00		✓ ✗ ↘
9:30		✓ ✗ ↘
10:00		✓ ✗ ↘
10:30		✓ ✗ ↘
11:00		✓ ✗ ↘
11:30		✓ ✗ ↘
12:00		✓ ✗ ↘
12:30		✓ ✗ ↘
1:00		✓ ✗ ↘
1:30		✓ ✗ ↘
2:00		✓ ✗ ↘
2:30		✓ ✗ ↘
3:00		✓ ✗ ↘
3:30		✓ ✗ ↘
4:00		✓ ✗ ↘
4:30		✓ ✗ ↘
5:00		✓ ✗ ↘
5:30		✓ ✗ ↘
6:00		✓ ✗ ↘

Top Energy Uses Today

Description	✓

What's Due

Rank	Task	🖋
		✓ ✗ ↘
		✓ ✗ ↘
		✓ ✗ ↘
		✓ ✗ ↘
		✓ ✗ ↘

Values Statement

Today I aligned my energy with my values by _____
_____
_____.

Good Things of Today

- ♥
- ♥
- ♥

Eat, Drink & Burn

Breakfast	
Lunch	
Dinner	
Snacks	

▢ ▢ ▢ ▢ ▢ ▢ ▢ ▢ Fitness:

ADDITIONAL RESOURCES

APA website with anxiety definition

1. American Psychological Association, 2020. apa.org/topics/ anxiety

2. Inspire More Blog by Scott Mautz, used with permission:https:// www.inspiremore.com/avoid-number-1-regret-of-dying/? utm_content=buffere2f4a&utm_medium=social&utm_source=f acebook.com&utm_campaign=IM

3. Lee, Richard B.; Daly, Richard Heywood (1999). **Cambridge Encyclopedia of Hunters and Gatherers.** Cambridge University Press. p. inside front cover. ISBN 978-0521609197. (https:// source.wustl.edu/2005/02/early-humans-were-prey-not-killers/)

4. Csikszentmihalyi, Mihaly. **Flow**: The Psychology of Optimal Experience. New York: Harper & Row, 1990._

5. Gladding, S. T., & Drake Wallace, M. J. (2018). Scriptotherapy: Eighteen Writing Exercises to Promote Insight and Wellness. Journal of Creativity in Mental Health, 13(4), 380-391.

6. Chapter Five - A helpful place to start is www.pandaplanner.com or www.happyplanner.com. These have great templates and ways to personalize your pages to your own needs. Alternately you can listen to or watch "Leaves on a Stream," which can be found at: https://www.youtube.com/watch?v=r1C8hwj5LXw

7. Chapter Seven - The website www.yourlifeyourvoice.org is one of my favorites. It lets you create a list of prompts based on themes.

ABOUT THE AUTHOR

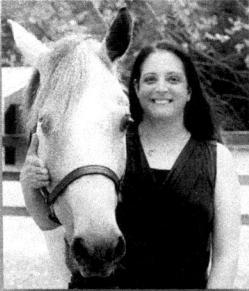

Cheryl is the founder of Mane Source Counseling and one of the founders of Horses and HEALTH Inc.

Her love of being around horses started very young, when she used to catch rides on ponies at her aunt's farm. At age ten, her grandmother Elsie bought her a horse of her own. She worked off her horse's expenses by cleaning stalls, feeding horses, and teaching lessons all the way through college. Before getting her masters in Counseling, Cheryl was a professional horse trainer, instructor and intercollegiate coach for over twenty years.

During her Masters studies at Bridgewater State University, Cheryl started working with a mentor in equine assisted counseling. After moving to North Carolina, she obtained her PhD from East Carolina University and started Mane Source. Her research interests are in equine assisted activities with clinical populations and with counselor supervision.

She facilitates Wellness Coaching for Stress Reduction, Supervision and Consultation for counselors, and continuing education workshops at the farm. When she's not working, her two boys, Christopher and Austin, keep her very busy!

Visit her website at
www.CherylMeola.com